CONQUERING DEPRESSION

A Guide to Understanding Symptoms, Causes, and Treatment of Depressive Illness

RUSSELL T. JOFFE, MD

ANTHONY J. LEVITT, MD

1998

Empowering Press, Hamilton, Canada

Canadian Cataloguing in Publication Data

Joffe, Russell T. 1954 —
   Conquering depression:

Includes index.
ISBN 0-9697781-7-1

1. Depression, Mental.   I. Levitt, Anthony J.,
1959 —   II. Title.
RC537.J64 1996   616.85′27   C95-933187-5

For distribution information contact the publisher:
Empowering Press
20 Hughson Street South, P.O. Box 620, L.C.D. 1
Hamilton, Ontario, Canada, L8N 3K7
Tel: 905-522-7017; Fax: 905-522-7839; e-mail: info@bcdecker.com;
Website: http://www.bcdecker.com   00 01 02/PC/65432

The authors and publisher have made every effort to ensure that the patient care recommended herein, including choice of drugs and drug dosages, is in accord with the accepted standards and practice at the time of publication. However, since research and regulation constantly change clinical standards, the reader is urged to check the product information sheet included in the package of each drug, which includes recommended doses, warnings, and contra-indications. This is particularly important with new or infrequently used drugs. Any treatment regimen, particularly one involving medication, involves inherent risk that must be weighed on a case by case basis against the benefits anticipated. The reader is cautioned that the purpose of this book is to inform and enlighten; the information contained herein is not intended as, and should not be employed as, a substitute for individual diagnoses and treatment.

Printed in Canada.

CONTENTS

DEDICATION

To our wives who provide unending support, and our children who provide unending joy.

Depression is much more than a feeling or emotion. It has the potential to be a severe and disabling mental illness with the potential to interfere with all aspects of a person's daily life. Although major depression is common, affecting about one in five people at some time in their lives, a great deal of misunderstanding exists about the nature of the illness and its diagnosis and treatment.

During the last 10 years, a lot has been learned about depressive illness and about its development and symptoms. Today, we know more about how this illness affects people—patients, family members, and friends. We know how depressive illness can influence lives. Better skills, techniques, and medications have been developed to treat it. *Today, most people who are clinically depressed can be successfully managed with*

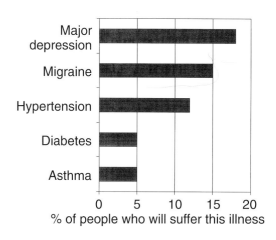

The risk of developing an illness during your lifetime

Depression is among the most common medical illnesses

antidepressant medications, some kinds of psychotherapy, or other treatment.

We wrote this book to inform you, and all people who are clinically depressed, about the dramatic advances that have been made in dealing with this disease. We wanted to explain how you, your family members, and/or your friends may take an active part in helping to manage and treat depressive illness successfully. We also wrote the book to clear away some of the confusion and misunderstanding about depressive illness that unfortunately still remains.

We hope you will find this book helpful. It is not meant to be a substitute for treatment; rather, what we tried to write was a handy source of information.

Russell T. Joffe, MD
Anthony J. Levitt, MD

CHAPTER 1

WHAT IS DEPRESSION?

Depression means different things to different people. A feeling of depression may be your reaction to things that occur in daily life. In some people, however, a feeling of depression can be a symptom—an indication—of an illness. Sometimes a medical condition such as anemia or thyroid disease can trigger a depressed mood. Even a common cold or "flu" can make some people feel down and blue.

Depression may also occur as a side effect of a medication you may have been prescribed. For example, beta-blocking drugs, which are prescribed for high blood pressure, may sometimes cause a patient to develop a depression.

In this book, however, we shall be discussing the most important meaning of the word "depression": depression as a distinct illness. This kind of depression is called "clinical depression" or "major depression."

There are many types of depressive illness; the most common is major depressive illness. This type of illness can be distinguished from other feeling states in three important ways. The distinguishing features of depressive illness are:

- The persistence and consistency of symptoms that last for more than 2 weeks. These symptoms affect a person almost all day, virtually every day.
- The connection with associated symptoms, e.g., emotional symptoms, physical symptoms, and altered or disordered thinking.
- The experience of dysfunction. Major depression can impair a person's ability to function normally in social situations, with other family members, and with people at work.

Symptoms of Depression

Emotional Symptoms

A depressed mood is the central symptom of major depression and occurs in almost 99% of patients. Many words and phrases are used to describe the emotional symptoms: "sad," "blue," "low," "lousy," "down-in-the-dumps," are just a few examples. If you are in your teens, nearing retirement, or retired, your major symptom may manifest as irritability, rather than a depressed mood. Surprisingly, the more and more depressed you become, the less likely you are to complain about your symptoms.

Anhedonia is a lack of interest in normally pleasurable activities. It is another primary symptom in major depression. A depressed person does not feel enthused about any activity (Table 1–1). Even if something does pique an interest, you do not enjoy doing it. Loss of sexual desire is another component of this symptom, and this sometimes results in a loss of sexual function that can be very disruptive. Not only does it deepen a low

Decreased Interest
• Someone with decreased interest might say one or more of the following about an activity that used to bring them pleasure: —"I just don't have the desire to do that any more"   —"I can't get motivated to do it"   —"Even though I want to do it, I can't get started"   —"Even though I get going with it, I can't seem to keep my interest in it. I can't seem to finish things"   —"Even though I get things done, I don't find any pleasure or satisfaction at having done it"   —"Even though I get things done, I don't look forward to trying again."

Table 1–1: The more depressed you become, the less likely you are to complain about your symptoms and the less likely you are to feel enthused about any activity.

mood but it can worsen existing difficulties in the relationship if you are married or involved in another intimate relationship.

Loss of sexual desire or function is a symptom very few people are able to discuss comfortably. However, sexual dysfunction can lead to the permanent break-up of a marital or long-term relationship. Whenever a couple complains about a loss of sexual function, doctors and other healthcare professionals look for signs and symptoms of depression in both partners.

Both these major symptoms—depressed mood and anhedonia—are persistent and consistent throughout a depressive episode, which will last for at least 2 weeks. During a depressed episode, these symptoms are present, not just for 1 or 2 hours but for almost all the hours of each day.

Physical Symptoms

If you have a major depressive illness you may also experience physical symptoms. You may find your appetite is less or, you may feel like eating too much. You may lose or gain weight, perhaps as much as 10 or more pounds. A reduction in appetite and body weight is a very common symptom in depressive illness.

Sleep can be disrupted. You may have trouble falling asleep, or staying asleep (Fig. 1–1). You may awaken at two or three in the morning and not be able to get back to sleep. (This will likely make your depressed mood worse; while all around are sleeping, you are awake, feeling lonely and isolated.) Even if you do sleep, you may wake up feeling tired—as if you had not slept at all. There are exceptions, however, and you may be one of them. Some depressed patients may oversleep, as many as 10 to 12 hours each night.

Another common symptom of depression is fatigue. This may manifest as a feeling of reduced energy that makes you tired and listless, or it may take the form of a heavy, physical tiredness that comes upon you after a normal activity that

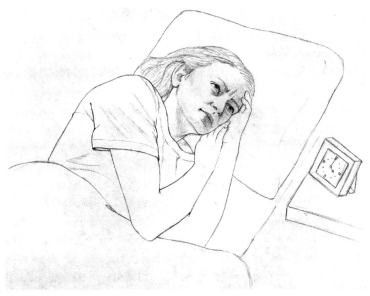

Figure 1–1: Sleep difficulties are a common and disabling feature of depression.

does not usually tire you at all. If you are depressed and have this symptom, even walking to the corner store may be exhausting.

Cognitive Symptoms

Altered thinking is a symptom that can range from mild to severe. A change in how efficiently you think may occur (Fig. 2A and B). You may lose the ability to concentrate or you may not be able to remember something that has just happened. Forgetting where you left your keys, for example, is something that happens to all of us at one time or another. But if you are severely depressed, it seems to happen all the time.

Altered or disordered thinking leads to a tremendous loss in your ability to function, especially at work. In the United States, it is estimated that business and industry lose more

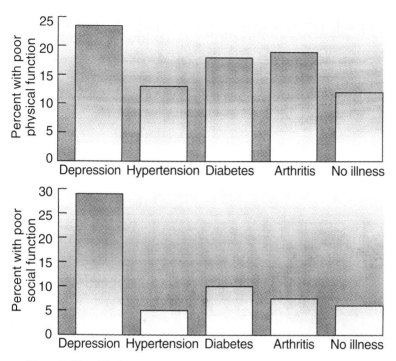

Figure 1–2A and B: Both physical and social functioning can be impaired during a depressive episode. *A*, shows how physical functioning is lowered in depression compared to other illnesses and *B*, shows how social functioning is impaired compared to the same illnesses in *A*.

than 10 billion ($U.S.) every year because of the reduction in efficiencies caused by major depressive illness.

Another change that can occur in depressive illness is more dangerous and ominous. You may feel excessively guilty, pessimistic, and have little or no self-esteem. You may feel helpless and hopeless. And being without hope, you may think of taking your own life. These thoughts lead to action in all too many cases; depression and/or alcohol are involved in 85% of all suicide attempts and deaths.

One important fact is worth noting and remembering. The belief that people who talk about committing suicide

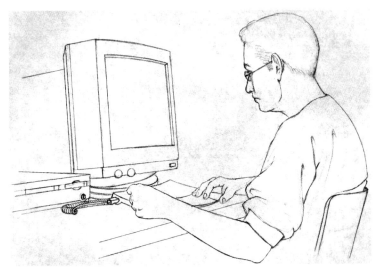

Figure 1–3: Problems with concentration and memory often lead to difficulties in daily life, especially in one's job.

will not do so is incorrect. *Most people who take their own lives speak of their intention before they act.*

Unfortunately, we cannot always predict which depressed individuals are most likely to take their own lives. However, if you have prepared a preventive plan of action, you can take steps to get help as soon as you realize that a change in your thinking is underway. And, as a relative or friend of a depressed person, there are things you can do to prevent a person from taking his or her own life. We discuss these in Chapter 10. There may be some consolation for all of us in the fact that suicides occur in only a very small percentage of the North American population.

You do not have to have all of the symptoms listed in Table 1-2 to be diagnosed as being depressed. However, if you have at least 5 of the 9 symptoms, and one of these is a

Table 1-2: Symptoms of Depression

Major Symptoms (Emotional)
    Depressed mood ("blue" gloomy, irritable)
    Anhedonia (complete loss of feeling in acts that usually give pleasure).
Secondary Symptoms
1. Cognitive
    Low self-esteem, excessive worry
    Reduced concentration or memory, trouble making decisions
    Thoughts of death
2. Physical
    Psychomotor changes (agitation, retardation)
    Decreased energy, fatigue
    Sleep changes, more or fewer hours of sleep
    Nutritional changes, increased or decreased appetite
    Gain or loss of body weight

major or emotional symptom (depression or anhedonia), you may be, by definition, clinically depressed.

Dysfunction

When depressed people are unable to take part in their usual social activities, their family life is disrupted, and they cannot work effectively at their jobs, they are said to be dysfunctional.

In a specific disorder or illness, when a number of signs and symptoms appear together, they are described as a syndrome (Fig. 1–4). When the syndrome occurs with dysfunction, this is the illness or disorder known as major depression.

People with depressive illness will have symptoms of other illnesses, too.

Anxiety

As many as one-third of depressed men and women will suffer from the clinical syndrome of anxiety during their lives, and up to 70% of people with an anxiety disorder will suffer from a major depressive episode at some point in their lives.

Depression as emotion, symptom and disorder

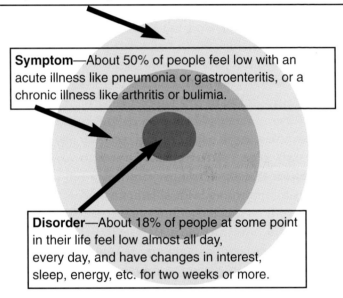

Emotion—Almost 100% of people feel low from time to time, for example, after a sad movie, when someone close moves away, or on hearing sad news.

Symptom—About 50% of people feel low with an acute illness like pneumonia or gastroenteritis, or a chronic illness like arthritis or bulimia.

Disorder—About 18% of people at some point in their life feel low almost all day, every day, and have changes in interest, sleep, energy, etc. for two weeks or more.

Figure 1–4: When a set of symptoms occur together, they are described as a syndrome. A major depression occurs when emotional symptoms cause dysfunction.

Depressed individuals may experience a range of anxiety symptoms. These can impact on emotional and physical well being or cause thinking to be altered or disordered as we have just described.

Emotional symptoms cause individuals to be overly anxious, worried, nervous, and vigilant. Physical symptoms originate from arousal of the autonomic nervous system which controls the involuntary activities of organs and other parts of the human body. The autonomic nervous system is overactive in most of the anxious patients. The overactivity makes the heart beat faster, the breathing rate change, and the stomach churn, and one may feel "sweaty" or "clammy."

Obsessions

A cognitive symptom of anxiety may take the form of obsessions. A depressed person may experience altered or disordered thinking. He or she may ruminate or think about the same negative subject over and over and over. It would not be unusual for a person with obsessions to think, "I am a failure; I'm useless; I'm hopeless"—again, again, and again.

Repetitive, unhelpful physical activity can make up the compulsive portion of the obsessional symptom. You may constantly wash your hands or shampoo your hair. Compulsions, too, may accord with the person's negative mood: "I am a bad person; I'm contaminated."

Panic Attacks

Another manifestation of the anxiety syndrome is physical: it takes on the form of a panic attack. Panic is the most intense form of anxiety any person can experience. Anxiety builds to such a peak that the patient may feel he or she is about to lose control. Some become terrified, believing they are about to die of a heart attack. These very disturbing attacks may last anywhere from a few minutes to an hour or more, but they are not life threatening.

Psychosis

A severe mental disorder where contact with reality is lost— psychosis—may also be part of the depression syndrome. Some patients have delusions (false beliefs that are not open to question and that are held fervently), which may also be consistent with the depressive syndrome. Patients suffering from a psychosis may believe they are nothing or have nothing (despite the contrary being true), or believe they are being unusually persecuted or that parts of their bodies are malfunctioning, dead, or rotting. Or, sufferers may have hallucinations, that is, sounds, images or sensations of things that do not actually exist; for example, they may hear voices that tell them they are worthless, or that they are nothing.

Symptoms of anxiety or psychosis can become so dramatic that, in some cases, they can mask a person's true illness. Only after carefully considering all the symptoms and the level of dysfunction they produce can a proper diagnosis of major depressive illness or of some other disease be made.

TYPES OF DEPRESSION

Psychiatrists classify major depression into several different categories. The first and most important distinction to be made is between unipolar and bipolar depression. The type of depression determines how it will be treated, what kind of advice you will receive, and how successful your treatment is likely to be.

Unipolar Depression

By far the most common type of major depression is of the unipolar type. Ninety percent of all people with a depression have this type. Episodes tend to last an average of 6 to 12 months. The number of symptoms required to diagnose a person with unipolar depression are listed in Table 1-2.

Bipolar Depression

Ten percent of depressed people suffer a bipolar depression— the depressive pole of manic depression or bipolar disorder. People with bipolar depression tend to exhibit a less common combination of symptoms, eating too much and oversleeping. The most important distinction between unipolar and bipolar depression is, however, the periods of mania (excitement or elation) that patients experience at the other pole of bipolar illness. Periods of mania are the hallmark of bipolar disorder. The treatment and course of bipolar depression are different from and somewhat more complicated than those for unipolar depression. Bipolar depression almost always requires the use of a mood-stabilizing drug. This book does not deal with the treatment of mania in its various presentations. This topic would need the writing of a whole other book.

Psychotic Depression

Psychosis occurs in 10% of depressed patients, of both bipolar and unipolar types. It may occur in only one episode of a series of six or seven nonpsychotic bouts, or a patient may experience psychotic depression every time depression strikes. Affected individuals have thoughts or beliefs that do not conform to reality. Thinking is very disorganized, and delusions may occur (fixed, irrational ideas with no basis in reality). Sometimes hallucinations are present (patients hear voices or sounds when none are present, or see things that other people do not see).

In psychotic depression, these delusions or hallucinations are "mood congruent." This means they harmonize with aspects of the patient's mood. For example, the unrealistic belief that someone wants to slight or harm them fits with symptoms of low self-esteem and feelings of worthlessness. The symptoms of psychosis, the delusions and hallucinations, do not usually persist after the depressive illness is cured. If they do, the diagnosis may have to be revised.

Schizophrenic individuals also have unreal thoughts and beliefs, but these bizarre symptoms commonly labelled "mood incongruent", because they may have nothing to do with what a person is actually feeling, are the central feature of the illness. (The belief that the television set is sending personal messages is an example of such an incongruent psychotic belief.)

Melancholic Depression

Melancholic depression is a very severe form of the illness and has many physical symptoms. Major symptoms are a significant loss of weight, awakening during the night, and complete loss of interest, enjoyment, and satisfaction in daily life. Men and women with this type of depression respond very well to antidepressants, electroconvulsive therapy (ECT), and to a lesser extent, psychotherapy.

Reactive and Endogenous Depression

Reactive depression is the name given to an episode of major depression that occurs after a specific life event. That event, sometimes called a trigger, can be a loss of any kind—person, job, pet, even a house. Reactive depression is common. It occurs in as many as 44% of all diagnosed depressions. Sometimes it is referred to as a situational or precipitated depression. Its opposite, endogenous depression, is one that emerges for no apparent reason.

People with reactive or endogenous depression present with the symptoms we described in Chapter 1. The symptoms and the syndromes in both these types of depression are the same. The duration and severity are also the same. When it comes to treatment, both reactive and endogenous depressions respond to psychotherapy and medication. Therefore, classifying depressions as endogenous or reactive is of limited use.

With respect to the treatment of reactive or endogenous depression, our strategy is just like the one physicians use to treat an attack of asthma. An asthma attack may be brought on by an allergen, by exercise, or even emotional stress. A doctor does not withhold medication just because the trigger of the attack has not been identified. Like an asthma attack, depression also occurs in episodes. These episodes must be treated, even if the trigger is unknown.

Some people report a clear relationship between a trigger and the onset of their illness. A closer look at events that preceded the depressive episode often reveals that symptoms of depression were in place before the suspected trigger was pulled. For example, a person may report that a problem that had occurred at work had precipitated the episode of depression; careful questioning may, however, reveal that the problem in the workplace had actually occurred because the person's concentration had been affected by a pre-existing depression and therefore his or her function at work.

Despite the fact that reactive and endogenous depressions have similarities for certain people, it is extremely helpful to the physician to understand what may precipitate a depressive episode. A person who gets depressed every time his or her family visits may need to take measures to avoid such visits or to plan with the therapist or psychiatrist for the visit.

Seasonal Depression

Seasonal depression, or seasonal affective disorder (SAD), occurs at a particular time of the year. Seasonal affective disorder is estimated to strike one in seven of all depressed individuals, or 2 to 4% of the general population (Fig. 2–1). It is a recurrent disorder that regularly emerges (usually during September to November) and also fades at a specific time of the year (usually March to May).

Why is SAD so regular in its appearance? Is it just because of the fewer daylight hours between fall and spring? Or do low

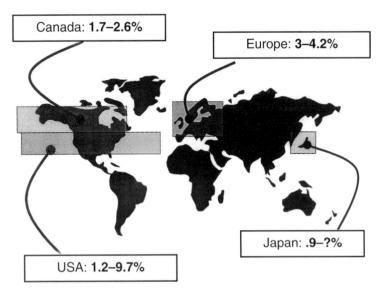

Canada: 1.7–2.6%

Europe: 3–4.2%

Japan: .9–?%

USA: 1.2–9.7%

Figure 2–1: Chances of having seasonal depression around the world.

winter temperatures, barometric pressure, and the amounts of precipitation have something to do with it? Although not proven, all of these are considered possible factors.

One bout of depression during winter does not mean you suffer from SAD. Not until you report two or three consecutive wintertime depressions do we begin to think of the likelihood of SAD. Then treatments are started, which may include light therapy or medication.

Anxious Depression

An anxious depression occurs when a general anxiety, phobia—a persistent fear—or panic are part of the illness. Forty percent of people with a major depression also suffer from an anxiety disorder at some time. Conversely, 70% of people with anxiety disorders will suffer from depression at some point in their lives. Frequently, people with major depression and anxiety disorder, share the same symptoms.

If anxiety is part of a depressive episode, it has a major impact on the overall situation. It not only increases the time it takes to become well, it reduces a person's long-term outcome. Also, the chances of a major depression occurring again are increased.

The good news is that if you receive adequate treatment for this type of depression and get well, you should be able to remain well. The critical factor is to get treatment as early as possible.

Minor Depression

The symptoms of minor depression are the same as those of major depression but are usually less severe and last for a long time. Dysthymia is a common type of minor depression and is categorized by chronic low-grade depression.

Dysthymia is less common than major depression, but dysthymic individuals seem predisposed to develop a major depression later on. The later development of a major depression is so likely that many of our colleagues believe dysthymia is a chronic risk condition for the development of major depression.

Double Depression

Double depression develops when the two disorders, major depression and dysthymia, occur at the same time in the same person. It can be compared to a patient suffering from asthma who develops bronchitis. With treatment, most people recover quickly from double depression, but recovery is not always complete. Although the major depression component of the disorder disappears, the dysthymia remains. Patients who have suffered from double depression also tend to relapse quickly into major depression.

Atypical Depression

Atypical depression is a subtype of depression that is distinguished by the patient's capacity to change moods as he or she reacts to events or activities. Physicians refer to this as "mood reactivity." Some people believe depressed men and women are "down" all the time, but this is not always the case. A patient can feel happy when good things happen, or feel worse when events are unhappy or bad. In both instances, however, the predominant mood is depression.

We diagnose a case as an atypical depression whenever we see mood reactivity with at least two of the following four symptoms: 1) increased eating; 2) increased sleeping; 3) an overly sensitive reaction (most often manifesting as a worsening of a depressed mood) to a real or perceived rejection; and 4) leaden fatigue.

The symptom of leaden fatigue is a preoccupation with physical feelings, usually a heaviness in the arms or legs.

Atypical depression is relatively uncommon but may more frequently be seen as part of a bipolar depression or seasonal depression.

How Common is Depression?

In the last 40 years, depression has become more common in North America. Currently, it is the most prevalent of all mental health disorders (Fig. 2–2). Two age groups account for most of this increase. The baby boomers, the men and women born in the late 1940s and early 1950s, and the second group, teenagers. The number of cases among this age group has risen significantly during the past 10 years. (Prevalence is usually expressed as the number of cases occurring per 100,000 people).

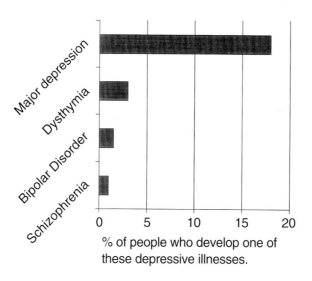

Figure 2–2: The risk of developing a depressive illness during a person's lifetime compared with risk of other common psychiatric illnesses.

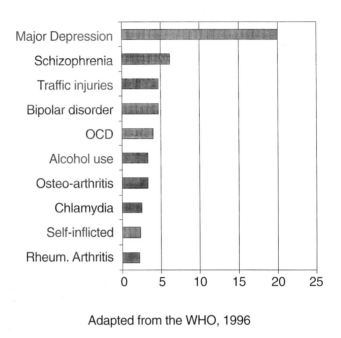

Adapted from the WHO, 1996

Figure 2–3: The ten leading causes of disease burden for women 15 to 45.

In North America, your chances of having a major depression are one in six during your lifetime. Put another way, at some point in life, 18% of the populations in the United States and Canada will have at least one episode of major depression in their lifetime. This contrasts with the incidence of diabetes or asthma which is around 5% (Fig. 2–3).

Seasonal affective disorder (SAD) will affect one in ten individuals, i.e., 2 to 4% of the population as a whole have SAD. An interesting finding is that, statistically, it may be quite normal to feel a little down during the winter period. In one study, 92% of people surveyed reported they had experienced one or more depressive symptom(s) that had proved more troublesome during the winter months. Difficulties included loss of energy, problems sleeping, and mood changes—all symptoms of depression. Although so many of us have difficulties with the winter months, especially in the more northerly climates, the number of persons with actual depressive illness is quite small.

You are more likely to suffer a major depression if you live in a city or metropolitan area. There may be several explanations for this phenomenon. In cities, people are more likely to experience the more intense stressors of daily life; or, perhaps, more health treatment services and facilities are available so that sufferers of depression may choose to live in cities in order to have access to private and public agencies that may provide financial and social support.

If you are a woman, you are more likely to suffer a major depression. Twice as many women than men experience an episode of major depression during their lives. For both men and women, however, the illness is most likely to emerge in the late to the mid-thirties. The incidence of bipolar depression is the same for both sexes. Although they may appear in younger children, bipolar symptoms frequently emerge in a mild form around age 15. The first visit to a health-care professional usually does not happen until the late teens. Then, it often takes another 4 to 5 years before a diagnosis of bipolar disorder is made, and still longer until treatment can be started.

Dysthymia is also slightly more prevalent among women.

Why do almost all types of depression affect more women than men? We do not know. One theory has a genetic basis: women are born with two X chromosomes, whereas men have only one X and one Y chromosome. If the disease is carried on the X chromosome, women would be more prone to depression. (Chromosomes contain genetic information that controls the activities of all human cells.) This theory has yet to be proved. According to another theory, different levels of some hormones in women account for the greater prevalence of depressive illness. Again, no convincing data have been produced.

Some experts believe that social factors are responsible for the difference between men and women in the incidence of depression. In the North American society, women are exposed to different stressors than men. For example, women with several children under the age of 10 and an absent husband are more likely to become depressed than are other women. Women, some say, were brought up to express their emotions more clearly than men. As children, women were also taught to seek help early when something was wrong. It could well be that each of these explanations and theories has some validity. Consideration of a combination of these factors may tell us why more women than men have periods of depression.

Depression occurs with almost equal frequency across all socioeconomic classes. Although there are more cases at the lower income levels, this does not mean that being poor is a cause of depression. It may show that illness impairs a person's capacity to earn.

The relationship between depression and unemployment is strong. As the unemployment rate increases in the general population, so does the number of new cases of major depressive illness. The suicide rate increases along with the rate of unemployment as well.

Marital status is also important in considering one's chances of becoming depressed as well as one's chances of recovery should illness occur. Married people are less likely to become depressed, but being married does not necessarily improve one's chances of recovery with treatment.

Depression leads to social impairment, producing conflict in relationships, the workplace, family life, studies, and leisure activities. What many people do not realize is that depression can also contribute to physical limitations. About half the people who suffer from depression also have some form of physical pain—be that headache, muscle pain, or back pain. Furthermore, in a study conducted in the United States, it was found that people with symptoms of depression could not climb stairs, walk, dress, or bathe as well as patients with other chronic medical conditions such as hypertension, arthritis, gastrointestinal problems, and back problems (see Fig. 1–2a).

Of concern to all healthcare professionals is that not all depressed men and women who seek treatment receive adequate therapy. Only 45% of people who are depressed actually seek treatment, and only half of them are believed to receive treatment. Furthermore, only half of this subgroup is treated successfully. What this means is that less than 10% of depressed men and women are getting adequate care.

A study was performed that rated treatments given to depressed patients at five major university-affiliated teaching hospitals. Barely 30% were judged to have received adequate therapy for their mood disorders—even, sometimes, in centers with experts in mood disorders!

Another study—this one done in Wales in the UK—looked at how general practitioners and family physicians prescribed antidepressant medications. More than half of them prescribed doses that were too low, and 40% prescribed them for periods that were too short to produce the optimal effect.

These poor results indicate a need to improve treatment for depression. More funding for undergraduate and continuing education would help. It is not that family physicians and psychiatrists receive poor training in medical school; rather, like everyone else, they are creatures of habit and tend to use the therapies most familiar to them. In this respect, psychiatrists and physicians are no different from other specialists who stay with the treatments they know best. More funding and more continuing medical education would certainly offset this situation. It should be noted, however, that updating of knowledge is now available not only to physicians but also to the general public. Information about depression, particularly, can be obtained in some Canadian provinces and the United States, toll-free, over the 1–888 lines.

Access to healthcare is another factor that impacts on the treatment of depression. Like many people working in other sectors of the economy, most of our colleagues are over-worked. The demand for psychiatric services in North America is not being met. Not enough practising psychiatrists are available, and those who are practising are not distributed evenly throughout the continent. Many rural and outlying areas of the United States and Canada do not have enough psychiatrists to serve the people living there. This is a healthcare problem that needs addressing.

Is Everyone Who Feels Blue Depressed?

The short answer is "No".

Only a very small percentage of people who feel miserable or "blue" are truly depressed. What separates people who always seem to feel low from those who are medically, or clinically, depressed is the syndrome described in Chapter 1. A certain set and number of symptoms plus significant dysfunction are indications of depression.

Nevertheless, a gray area separates feeling blue and being clinically depressed, the difference between a simple change in mood and a clinical syndrome. Making the distinction between the two is what psychiatrists and other doctors try to do when they first see a person who may be depressed.

For example, people who are always miserable—rude, nasty, irritable, personally isolated—are bound to have poor social relationships. Who, after all, wants such people as close friends? However, as we have seen, poor social relations may be one of the symptoms of depression. Are these people rude and irritable because they have few, if any, friends? Or, do they lack friends because of their negative hehavior or depressive episode?

A domestic dispute with a spouse or partner may be enough to trigger some symptoms of depression. After a quarrel, it is likely that you will not have much of an appetite.

You will probably lie awake most of the night and brood about what has happened. Life seems unfair and nobody seems to understand you. But the next day, life is back on an even keel, and the apparent symptoms of depression dissipate.

Many, otherwise healthy individuals experience mood swings that sometimes lack an explanation. Others, for understandable reasons, may become miserable at certain regular periods. Being short of money near the end of each month is a good enough reason for some to feel sad and be miserable for a few days. However, these are normal changes in mood, not signs of a depressive illness.

The reverse is also true. Even if you are suffering from a major depression, you may not be depressed every minute of every day of the year. You may sometimes enjoy periods when you feel happy and wear a wide smile on your face.

These are some of the reasons why a diagnosis of depression is not made until the syndrome—the group of symptoms *and* the dysfunctions that define depression—persists for at least 2 weeks.

Grief

Grief, or a loss, is a difficult experience to assess. Grief is a change in mood that occurs as a reaction to a significant loss. When someone loses a spouse or partner, or especially a child, grief can be profound. A loss can be felt so deeply that the syndrome of depression may emerge. The survivor feels sad, will not eat, cannot get a full night's sleep, and cannot concentrate at work.

This kind of grief is normal but only up to a point. After a certain period of time, it can become an illness—major depression. Unfortunately, we, and our colleagues, cannot always tell when a grieving survivor crosses the line between what is a normal reaction to loss and depressive illness.

At one time we thought the more severe the symptoms of grief initially, the better off the survivor would be in the long

Table 2-1: Indicators That Grief
May Have Turned Into Depression

- Grief persists beyond three months after the death
- Suicidal ideation (not just the philosophical desire to be with the deceased loved one)
- Past history of major depression
- Psychotic experiences (hallucination or delusions)
- Depressed mood apparent all day everyday, and associated with other symptoms of major depression for more than a month
- Decreased ability to care for self

term. Today, we think that "too little or too much" is what counts. Too little may mean the survivor is not dealing with his or her grief, and too much may indicate a true depression.

If, after about 3 months, the survivor of a loss still suffers from the syndrome of depression, medical treatment may be needed. By this time, a grieving person should be taking some steps to return to a normal daily life (Table 2–1).

We know profound grief is more likely in those who have a history of depression, and in those who have been in a relationship for many years. Depression is more common also in people who have experienced intense and conflict-ridden relationships. Survivors may feel guilty about what has been said or done to the deceased during the relationship. Deep, long-lasting grief is also more likely to occur in women. One explanation of this phenomenon is that women tend to outlive men in a marriage.

What should psychiatrists and doctors do for people who suffer profound grief after a major loss? The answer, in most cases, is to let them be. A medical condition should not be created from what is a very human reaction. Some grieving men and women think of taking their own lives, and they may express this wish. If we see this in a person who exhibits a very intense syndrome and who has a history of depression, we may want to treat it right away. Ten out of every 100 people who suffer a major loss require out-patient treatment at psychiatric clinics.

CHAPTER 3

CAUSES OF DEPRESSION

Depression is a complex illness with many causes. Although we cannot list the causes of depression, we can make some very informed guesses about what factors are to some degree responsible.

We know, for example, that depressive illness and manic depressive illness are basically disorders of the brain. Like a top rate orchestra whose musicians always play together to produce beautiful music, the human brain is a marvel of harmonious interaction. In depressive illness, however, the orchestra becomes unbalanced, its music off-key. The wind section plays something completely different from the strings, percussion different from brass. Some people refer to this disharmony as a "chemical imbalance."

There is good evidence to support that some genetic factors play a role in creating this imbalance.

We know, for example, that relatives of depressed individuals are more likely than other men and women to become depressed during their lifetimes. For the general public, the risk of becoming ill with depression at some point in life is between 17 and 20%. For first degree relatives—parents, children, brothers and sisters—there is a modest increase in this risk.

Studies of twins provide stronger evidence for a genetic factor. Twins can be either identical (monozygotic) or fraternal (dizygotic). Identical twins develop from a single ovum and share the same placenta. Each has exactly the same genetic material as the other. At birth they are of the same sex and look almost exactly alike.

Fraternal or nonidentical twins develop from separate ova, and each has its own placenta. Fraternal twins may be of the same or different sex, and they may not look alike. They have and share only the same amount of genetic material as would a brother or a sister.

Studies of twins reveal that if one identical twin develops depression, the other has a 60% chance of developing it. With nonidentical twins, the risk of one developing a depression after the first is only 15 to 25%—the same risk faced by other first-degree relatives.

These studies of twins, reveal two important pieces of information. First, people with identical genes have a greater chance of becoming depressed after one of the group becomes ill. We can, therefore, conclude that genetics must play a role. However, the second piece of information reveals that, since the likelihood of this happening is only 60%, a genetic factor cannot be the *only* one involved in predisposing a person to depression. Other factors must also play a role—even in cases of identical twins.

Stronger evidence to support the involvement of a genetic factor comes from Scandinavia. Scandinavian studies reveal that some children may carry their genetic predisposition to depression into an adoptive environment, even when that environment is otherwise free of depression.

What these studies show is that if children are born to parents with a history of depression but are adopted at birth by families free from depression, the children's risk of becoming depressed is still 15%. This is the same degree of risk faced by first-degree relatives.

In recent years, research into the genetic causes of disease has become a very important part of medical research (Table 3–1). Every cell in the human body has more than 50,000 genes in its nucleus, and each human being is composed of billions of cells. The focus of current research is on genes because they influence the chemical processes that go on in human cells. Through the cells, genes influence the operation of every human organ and system. Researchers believe that finding the gene responsible for a specific function or action will allow the identification of the chemical it influences. They hope to identify any abnormality in that chemical that may cause a particular disease. If there is an abnormality, and if it does cause disease, some way to correct the abnormality and prevent the disease may be found.

Common Illnesses That Have A Genetic Component
• Coronary Artery Disease • Bowel Cancer • Familial Alzheimer's Disease • Bipolar Disorder • Thalassemia • Sickle Cell Anemia • Depression

Table 3–1: Researchers believe that genetics could play a role in the development of depression.

The search for genes that may be involved in the development of depression is receiving a lot of attention. One current research project is trying to isolate the genes which may be involved in the development of manic depression.

In many respects, depression resembles diabetes. Diabetes develops when the pancreas fails to produce enough of the hormone insulin. Insulin moves glucose (sugar) to the inside of cells, which allows the production of energy in the cells. Lack of insulin means cells cannot receive enough glucose, which creates a chemical imbalance. Diabetics who are insulin dependent can restore this balance: they control their disease by taking injections of insulin. On their own, however, these injections are not enough. To maintain adequate control, diabetics must also eat a healthy diet, exercise regularly, and not smoke.

Unfortunately, we do not yet have an "insulin" for depression. But if, and when, we do, depressed individuals will still have to take other steps: proper diet, exercise, and other habits of healthy living.

Our ignorance about the chemicals which may be involved in depression is mainly a matter of developing the ability to identify specific ones. As many as 800 chemicals are involved in the functioning of the human brain—and more are discovered every year. Although we cannot pinpoint exactly those that may be involved in depression, three are suspected of playing a role: serotonin, norepinephrine, and dopamine.

Serotonin

This chemical is found in many parts of the body, including the neurons (nerve cells) of the brain, the digestive tract, and the platelets in the blood. Not all of the neurons in the brain contain serotonin. Those that do are located in discrete areas.

Serotonin acts as a neurotransmitter. Its job is to transmit nerve impulses or "messages" between certain cells in the nervous system. The pathways that these impulses move along affect some basic human functions. Serotonin pathways affect eating, sex drive, and physical movements. To a smaller degree these pathways may influence concentration and memory. They also affect the limbic system which is located in the center of the brain. The limbic system plays a role in regulating moods and emotions.

Identifying abnormalities in the levels of serotonin in the brain is not easy. Ethical considerations do not allow medical researchers to extract pieces of living brain for study. The alternative is to study the chemical itself, or its breakdown products. These can be found in the blood or urine, or in the cerebrospinal fluid that bathes the brain.

Although this method is not perfect, it has provided valuable information. We know, for example, that a link exists between low serotonin levels and a greater tendency to violence and suicide. This suggests that both violence and suicide have a biochemical, and possibly genetic, foundation.

Norepinephrine

Norepinephrine, which is also known as noradrenaline or adrenalin, is a hormone. This hormone is responsible, amongst other things, for regulating blood pressure. You may recognize it for the part it plays in the human fear response. Levels of adrenalin rise quickly when a person becomes anxious or frightened.

Relatively few neurons in the brain contain norepinephrine. They are closely related to the neurons that contain serotonin and those that are involved in the same physical and emotional functions. Like serotonin, noradrenaline can be found in other parts of the body, and it cannot be examined directly in the brain. It can only be measured indirectly. It is difficult to know what the current results of these measurements mean.

Levels of norepinephrine in depressed people are clearly abnormal. However, we are not sure as yet if levels are abnormally low or abnormally high. Most experts used to think it was too low. Today, however, medical and research opinion favours the view that in depression, levels are too high. Low or high, the evidence we have now suggests that some abnormality in the efficiency of the noradrenaline system is involved in the development of depression. This abnormality may be the cause of most of the physical symptoms of depression.

Dopamine

This neurotransmitter is found in some blood vessels as well as the brain. Dopamine helps control body movements. A deficiency of dopamine in the basal ganglia, which are deep inside the brain, causes Parkinson's disease; dopamine may also play some role in depression, particularly manic depressive illness, but its role is less clear than is the case with serotonin or norepinephrine.

Hormones

Hormones have also been linked to depression.

Many depressed people have underactive thyroid glands. Their glands produce low levels of thyroid hormones which help regulate the metabolism. Not all people with underactive thyroids are, however, clinically depressed although they may exhibit the symptoms. In fact, some people with overactive thyroid glands may exhibit symptoms of anxiety or depression. That is why thyroid function tests are often ordered when a doctor sees someone he or she suspects is suffering from depression.

There is also a link between the adrenal glands, which produce steroid hormones, and depression. Located above the kidneys, the small, triangular glands produce cortisone and cortisone-like substances called corticosteroids. These influence a number of important body systems and functions.

Hormones and chemicals in the body take part in the cascade of biological events linked with various causes of depression. Unfortunately, we still do not know how or where this chemical hormone flow begins. Do the chemicals prompt the hormones into action or is it the other way around? We may eventually learn that other factors, as yet unknown, are involved in this process.

Life Events

When a depressive illness occurs, psychological and social factors also appear to be involved. Bereavement, loss of a job, financial difficulties, and other adverse events will not on their own cause a depression, but they may make you more vulnerable to the illness if you also have the genetic and biochemical predisposition.

Early life events are known to produce major depressive illness years later. More than a few depressed people lost their mothers before they were 17 years old. This loss may have altered the body chemistry of these people in some as yet unknown way, thereby making them candidates for depression.

Some factors are more immediate. These factors are more likely to be physical and psychological. Some patients, for example, report a severe bout of flu or a trauma like a broken leg or surgery just before a period of depression started.

Several psychological theories have been put forward to explain the onset of depression. One is known as the cognitive theory. This theory holds that if you think in certain negative ways you may become depressed. One cognitive model of depression, developed 25 years ago, led to a successful treatment. The treatment is known as cognitive behaviour therapy. It is based upon the belief that a person becomes depressed because he or she thinks in a negative fashion about him or herself, the surrounding world, and the future. This is referred to as the cognitive triad—self, world, future.

Another model of depression, the learned helplessness model, suggests that if nothing in life turns out as it should, the person learns to respond to each setback in everyday life by becoming depressed.

In yet another model, depression is thought to be a reaction to living in a tough, unequal world. A component of this model is based on the observation that more women than men become depressed because modern life is still lived in a "man's world."

Biological Rhythms

Most biological organisms—including human beings—attempt to organize and adjust their lives according to a regular rhythm. And for the most part, the attempt is successful. Humans like to follow a daily pattern for nourishment, activity, and rest—three meals a day, and one wake and one sleep period. If we have to live through four seasons, we make the necessary practical and biological adjustments for the heat of the summer and the cold of the winter.

Some psychiatrists have shown that in depressed individuals these normal biologic rhythms are disrupted. A depressed person's sleep-wake cycle is not synchronised; it does not follow a normal rhythm. This, in turn, disrupts other biochemical processes, and as a result, these individuals become depressed.

It is interesting to note that while humans keep time with their biological rhythms quite well, their bodies cannot exactly follow the 24-hour cycle devised to account for night and day. Our biological rhythms work on a cycle of 24.5 or 25 hours. A slight discrepancy exists, and we have to correct this out-of-sync rhythm. We do this by responding to environmental cues.

Sunrise and sunset, eating meals at fairly regular intervals, and leaving for and returning from work at the same time are just some of the daily factors that are used to alter and retrain our biological rhythms.

Drug Abuse

Alcohol and drug abuse or addiction are believed to be implicated in the emergence of depression. In a recent study, 70% of people who entered an alcohol and drug rehabilitation program were diagnosed as suffering from a major depression. Although none was treated for depression, after the rehabilitation program was successfully completed, only 4% still suffered from major depressive illness.

These findings should not come as a surprise. If taken in excess over an extended period of time, alcohol acts like a poison on the brain. There is no doubt that alcohol affects the synapses and neurotransmitters that are involved in determining a person's moods and in transporting and processing the antidepressant drugs used to treat mood disorders.

At first glance, you may wonder if these different theories about causes of depression are exclusive or if they compete with one another. The biochemist may say—with very good authority—that depression is caused by a chemical abnormality. The psychologist may claim that depression is the result of negative thinking that has become a habit. The

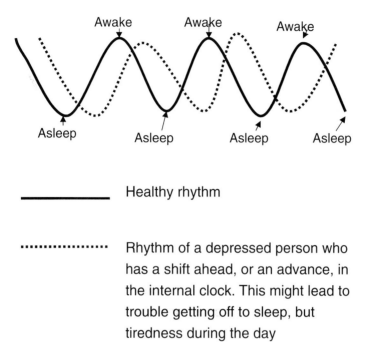

Awake   Awake   Awake

Asleep   Asleep   Asleep   Asleep

_____ Healthy rhythm

················ Rhythm of a depressed person who has a shift ahead, or an advance, in the internal clock. This might lead to trouble getting off to sleep, but tiredness during the day

Figure 3–1: In a depressed person, the normal internal clock may be disrupted.

psychotherapist may tell you that depression is a reaction to events that have taken place in your past life. In fact, all of these theories may be mutually inclusive or mutually supporting because the brain is involved in all these areas.

Whatever turns out to be the one explanation, there is no doubt that as human beings, we interact in an exquisitely complex way with our environment. This interaction is so tight and multifaceted that it is extremely difficult to distinguish between the functions of human cells, brain chemistry, and the environment.

CHAPTER 4

DIAGNOSTIC TESTS FOR DEPRESSIVE ILLNESS

If you think you may be suffering from some form of depression, there are three available sources of confirming whether a diagnosis of depression is right or wrong: yourself; a psychiatrist, family physician, or other doctor; and a close friend or a member of your family.

Yourself

Begin by evaluating your present situation. Ask yourself these questions: Have I felt sad, blue, miserable, or gloomy for a while recently? Have I lost interest in doing things I usually enjoy? If the answer is "Yes" to either, or both, of these questions, there is a chance that you could be depressed in some way.

Another option is to complete the check list provided in Table 4-1. The Beck Depression Inventory provides a means of measuring a person's level of depression. Psychiatrists may use it when talking with a patient for the first time. This scale, and others like it, do not diagnose depression, but they determine how severe it is. What is your symptom score? If you score more than 15 or 16, there is, again, a good chance you may be suffering from depression; so, consult your family physician.

Learning about a disease is a way to find out if you have the syndrome that defines an illness. Reading this book is an example of an attempt to determine whether or not you are depressed. Another option is to contact a self-help group or other volunteer organization such as the Canadian Mental Health Association. Groups like these usually have literature available. Some even have counselors you can talk with on the telephone or in person. You can also visit your local library or book store.

If you have some of the more severe symptoms of depression—poor concentration, low self-esteem, loss of energy—these may prevent you from taking any of these steps. Like

Table 4–1   For at least a two week period have you...
☑ been feeling down or low or blue almost every day
☑ lost interest in things that you used to enjoy
☑ lost energy, feeling physically tired or fatigued
☑ had trouble concentrating, or making decisions
☑ been feeling agitated or restless, or feeling very sluggish or slowed down
☑ been thinking about death or wanting to die, or feeling life isn't worth living
☑ been very worried, or feeling guilty about things you have no control over or didn't do
☑ had trouble sleeping, or been oversleeping
☑ lost your appetite or had weight loss, or been overeating or had weight gain
virtually all day?
Total 2 or less—unlikely major depression, but may have other health problem
Total 3—unlikely major depression, but still may benefit from visit to family doctor for assessment
Total 4 (one is either depressed mood or lost interest)—likely depression, see your doctor
Total 5 (one is either depressed mood or lost interest)—High likelihood of depression, see your doctor immediately

other depressed individuals, you may not realize or accept that you are suffering from an illness. When you are depressed, it can be difficult even to try to learn how and why you feel the way you do. Do what you can. People with these symptoms may tend to blame themselves. They may make an attempt to find out more about why they feel the way they do but are not up to completing the task. When these people start to feel better, they may, however, be able to concentrate more efficiently and retain more information. It is worthwhile to find out what you need to know about major depression when you are well.

Psychiatrist or Family Doctor

Going to see your family physician, a psychiatrist, or a psychiatric healthcare worker is a productive step. However, not all family doctors or healthcare workers can recognize the

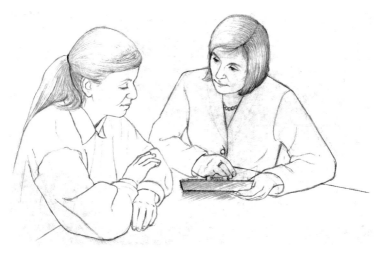

Figure 4–1: Your family physician or psychiatrist will do a "workup" during your first visit.

more subtle forms of depression. If you feel that is the case in your situation, get a second opinion from another family doctor or from someone working in the psychiatric field.

When you see either a family physician or a psychiatrist for the first time, he or she will do what is called a "work up" (Fig. 4–1). This involves taking a short history of your life, giving you a physical examination, and perhaps taking a blood sample which would be needed for tests (e.g., a thyroid function test).

Your first visit to a family physician will probably not result in definite answers about your illness. Your visit will probably last only 20 minutes. At this time, the goal is to look for other possible causes of your mood changes. If everything is normal—including blood test results that usually arrive a few days later—the doctor will then start to consider what form of depression you may be suffering from. A discussion of possible treatments may begin at this time.

If you are first seen by a psychiatrist, the visit may last as long as 45 minutes to an hour. The psychiatrist will make a diagnosis after considering five factors:

1. **Presentation:** What you are currently experiencing and how you describe your present situation.
2. **Personal History**: Has this ever happened to you before? Has it been going on for some time?
3. **Family History**: Does anyone in your family—present and past—have a history of some form of a psychiatric illness, particularly of anxiety, depression, or drug/alcohol abuse?
4. **Biological markers:** As yet, blood tests cannot diagnose depression. The tests that may be performed at this time are used to exclude other illnesses that may produce depressive symptoms.
5. **Treatment response**: How a patient responded to a specific treatment in the past sometimes helps make a diagnosis of major depression.

Some psychiatrists will give you a questionnaire to fill out, similar to the Beck Depression Inventory (see Table 4-1). The Hamilton Rating Scale, which has an interview format, is probably the best known tool for evaluating depression. The interview (or scale) allows a physician to evaluate the severity of a depression. It has been used for over 30 years but is usually only used by researchers.

Interviews, tests, and questionnaires do not absolutely guarantee a diagnosis. Healthcare workers, being human, sometimes make mistakes. However, when we see the syndrome that defines depression, along with dysfunctional behaviour, we can be sure that something is amiss.

We also know that if a patient is not suffering from a sickness such as anemia or thyroid disease, and has presented with symptoms of depression, there is a very high chance of the illness being a major depression. One should remember that depression is a treatable illness, even when other illnesses are not. In cases where the diagnosis of the presenting illness is uncertain, it sometimes is a good idea to go ahead and consider treating the illness as depression anyway. Even when the initial diagnosis is depression, the clinician or therapist should always keep in mind that it may be some other medical condition.

Even professionals other than psychiatrists may be able to help you onto the road to early diagnosis and successful treatment. Many patients we see for the first time are suffering from a depression they did not recognize. They are referred to us by social workers, psychologists, occupational therapists, priests, ministers, and rabbis. Many of these professionals have had some mental healthcare training, or specialize in mental health, and may have developed counseling skills. They can, therefore, be very astute at recognizing the symptoms of depression. It is worthwhile listening to them if they suspect depression.

Family and Friends

Members of the immediate family are usually the first people to notice changes in another family member's mood and behavior. You may, however, hesitate to approach members of your family because you may feel ashamed or frightened of being told you are sick. Your concerns could be valid; their response may be that you "get off the couch and get on with something."

These reactions on the part of family members are normal. Your brother, sister, or parent may find it difficult to recognize and accept that you are ill. They may find it more comforting to believe you would indeed get better if you just got busy and did something.

It is a good idea, then, to ask someone in your family who is not likely to be judgmental and who will respond to you in a helpful way. You may find that you need to speak to more than one person to get a balanced, yet candid, view of your situation. Perhaps you do not consider that you can get a balanced opinion in your family. If this is the case, consider other candidates: a very close friend, a fellow employee, or even a very understanding boss. Whoever you approach, it is important that you believe you have their trust and that they will respect your confidence.

The idea of hospitals and clinics, and even a doctor's office worries some people. If you are one of these, it is a good idea to talk with a family member first or with a friend connected to the healthcare system. If you do have such a friend, he or she may be able to tell you what to expect from the system and, thereby, reduce your worries and fears.

The important thing to remember is that you are *not* responsible for your illness. Like diabetes and Alzheimer's disease, depression is an illness that befalls you. You are not responsible for that or to blame. Your only responsibility is to get treatment and, once this has begun, to stay with the therapy until you are well again.

How Healthcare Professionals Test for Depression

If they wish, psychiatrists and other professionals can refer to manuals and other references when they first interview and examine a person for a possible depression. These types of reference materials list the primary and secondary signs and symptoms of illness. Definitions and/or criteria are incorporated into various questionnaires that you may be given during interviews. Most experienced clinicians know the symptoms well and do not need to refer to manuals.

A major depression can be diagnosed without these diagnostic manuals. A 10- to 15-minute across-the-desk interview is often enough for a trained mental health worker to decide if the person is seriously depressed, or if some other malady is responsible. Some types of depression, however, may require a longer interview, perhaps 45 to 90 minutes before a decision can be made.

Bipolar illness can often be diagnosed without recourse to the structured interview. This is because the illness always exhibits episodes of mania which are easy to recognize. However, some forms of bipolar disorder may be missed entirely unless mental health workers are alert to the subtle symptoms or are aware of the possible subtypes of depression. In these cases, structured interviews and reference manuals can be of great assistance.

The Diagnostic and Statistical Manual of Mental Disorders— referred to as DSM-4 because it is in its fourth edition—is a valuable reference often consulted by psychiatrists. This manual organizes the descriptions of the signs and symptoms of mental illnesses in sections and ascribes codes for each one. The codes are sometimes required by insurance companies so that there is a standardized way of communicating the physician's diagnosis.

Using the DSM-4 allows a psychiatrist to make a diagnosis that helps to develop a pretty good idea of what treatment to use first and indicates how good the chances for a successful outcome are. The DSM-4 is important for another reason: it helps to ensure that psychiatrists and others always "talk the same language."

It is essential that as many of the symptoms of depression are recorded. This way, the progress of your illness can be monitored. For, unlike a blood test for anemia or a pulmonary function test for asthma, no single laboratory or other test can be used to diagnose a mood disorder. The change in the severity of symptoms is our only gauge.

CHAPTER 5

HOW ANTIDEPRESSANTS WORK

How the various classes of antidepressant drugs work we cannot exactly say, but how they affect the cells of the central nervous system is well known. We know that antidepressants do work because we see the results in our depressed patients.

The first antidepressant drugs were discovered by chance and good luck almost 40 years ago. The first category of antidepressants, the monoamine oxidase inhibitors (MAOIs), were originally used to treat tuberculosis (TB). Monamine oxidase inhibitors did not always cure or stop the advance of TB, but physicians noticed that tubercular patients were in a better mood when they took these drugs. Some patients even became manic while taking them.

The second category of drugs, the tricyclic antidepressants (TCAs), were also developed in the late 1950s. More recently, two other categories of drugs have become available: the selective serotonin reuptake inhibitors (SSRIs). Serotonin reuptake inhibitors were introduced in 1989 and the serotonin-norepinephrine reuptake inhibitors (SNRIs) in the mid-1990s. Also in the mid-1990s, the reversible inhibitor of monoamine oxidase A (RIMA's) were released to the market. These different classes of antidepressants work in different ways. The different categories of antidepressants available by decade are shown in Fig. 5–1.

Tricyclic Antidepressants

At first these drugs were thought to work by stopping the reuptake of serotonin and adrenalin. Simply put, tricyclics would slow the return of these neurotransmitters back into the neurons that originally stimulated their release into the synapse. (A synapse is the site between neurons where impulses are transmitted from one neuron to the other by electrical or chemical means.) Blocking the reuptake increases the amount of serotonin and adrenalin floating in the

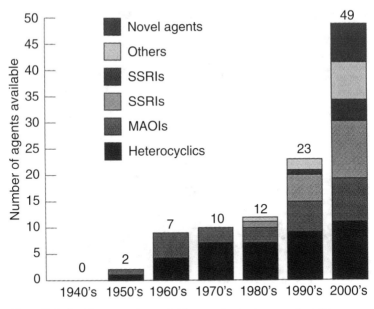

Figure 5–1: Antidepressants available over the last seven decades.

synapse, thereby making more of these neurotransmitters available at the receptor sites. This is how the tricyclics were thought to combat the low levels of serotonin that most doctors used to think caused depression.

This explanation fits nicely with the older theories of depression. However, the explanation is now open to debate. So far, evidence is not available to support the theory that low levels of serotonin and/or norepinephrine is the sole cause of changes in mood. Furthermore, even people who do not get better have the reuptake successfully blocked.

There is no doubt that a dose of imipramine—the first tricyclic to be developed—will begin to block the reuptake of both serotonin and norepinephrine within a few hours. However, if blocking reuptake were all that was necessary for the antidepressants to work, one would expect the patient to feel better as soon as the blockage occurred. This is not what actually happens. It takes 3 to 4 weeks before imipramine has any effect on a person's mood.

The delay between biochemical action and clinical effect has stimulated debate among researchers and doctors. There is no agreement that blocking the reuptake of neurotransmitters is the critical mode of action of the tricyclics in depression.

Monoamine Oxidase Inhibitors

After their release, norepinephrine and serotonin are broken down by the enzyme monoamine oxidase. The inhibitor of monoamine oxidase (an MAOI) prevents this breakdown. By doing so, a backup of serotonin and norepinephrine is created in the synapse, thereby raising the level of both neurotransmitters. However, is this the main mode of action? Again, no one knows.

The enzyme, monamine oxidase, is required by the body to break down a substance called tyramine. The MAOI, therefore, prevents the body from destroying tyramine which is found in a variety of foods. However, if tyramine is not destroyed, it may cause rapid increase in blood pressure. For this reason, people being treated with MAOIs must adhere to a specific "MAOI diet." A list of the currently available antidepressant medications is given in Table 5–1. However, recently the RIMAs have been developed. These are similar to the MAOIs except they do not require dietary restriction. If someone on an RIMA (moclobemide is the only one currently available) they do not have to avoid tyramine-rich food—unlike people taking older MAOIs.

Selective Serotonin Reuptake Inhibitors

These medications are very popular. They are selective because they affect predominantly the reuptake of serotonin. The older antidepressants such as the TCAs or the older MAOIs not only block serotonin and/or norepinephrine but

Table 5-1: Antidepressant Medications

Class	Chemical Name	Brand Name	Usual Starting Dose (mg)	Usual Dose (mg per day)	Dose Range (mg)
SSRIs	Fluoxetine	Prozac	20	20	5–80
	Fluvoxamine maleate	Luvox	50	100	50–300
	Sertraline HCl	Zoloft	50	100	50–200
	Paroxetine HCl	Paxil	20	20	20–60
TCAs	Imipramine HCl	Tofranil	40	150*	50–300
	Amitriptyline HCl	Elavil	50	150*	50–300
	Desipramine HCl	Norpramin	50	150*	50–300
	Nortriptyline HCl	Aventyl	25	75†	50–100
	Doxepin HCl	Sinequan	50	150	50–200
	Trimipramine HCl	Surmontil	50	150*	50–300
	Clomipramine HCl	Anafranil	50	150*	50–300
	Maprotiline HCl	Ludiomil	50	150	50–300
	Protriptyline HCl	Triptil	10	30	30–60
	Amoxapine HCl	Asendin	50	150	15–300
	Trazodone HCl‡	Desyrel	50	200	100–400
RIMAs	Moclobemide	Manerix	150	600§	450–900
MAOIs	Tranylcypromine	Parnate	10	60§	30–90
	Phenelzine sulphate	Nardil	15	75§	60–120
SNRIs	Nefazodone HCl	Serzone	150	450§	300–600
	Venlafaxine HCl	Effexor	75	225§	150–300
Other	Bupropion HCl	Wellbutrin	76	300§	75–450

*Daily dose is determined using the following formula: 2.5 × your body weight in kilograms; †dose is determined by blood level testing; ‡Trazodone not really a tricyclic antidepressant, but it has similar profile so is included in this section; §Should be given in divided doses, (i.e., two or three times a day).

also tend to affect other neurotransmitters. This results in no added benefit but lots of side effects. Once again, we know that this action takes place, but we do not know if this is the critical step in relieving symptoms of depression.

The SSRIs were developed specifically to block the reuptake of serotonin. They have little effect on other receptors and systems. There are fewer side effects with the SSRIs than with the older antidepressants. The RIMAs also have fewer side effects.

The tricyclics, on the other hand, affect many other receptors and systems in the body. This explains some of their side effects such as dry mouth, blurred vision, a bloated feeling in the stomach, among others.

Serotonin-Norepinephrine Reuptake Inhibitors

Known as SNRIs or mixed reuptake inhibitors, the two drugs available in this class selectively stop the reuptake of both serotonin and norepinephrine. One of these, venlafaxine, may work better as its dose is increased. Therefore, people who can tolerate high doses are most likely to achieve the greatest benefit. The other, nefazodone, has only a very small effect on the reuptake of serotonin and norepinephrine, but it does have a direct effect on receptor sites; it imitates a neurotransmitter in the synapse and actually blocks the effect of the neurotransmitters.

Lithium

This drug is the treatment of choice in bipolar depression. Lithium, alone, is about as effective as a placebo in cases of unipolar illness.

Other Antidepressants

Bupropion blocks the reuptake of dopamine, yet another neurotransmitter. This drug is among the least likely to affect a person's sexual desire or function. In high doses, however, it has a higher risk than most other drugs of inducing seizures in people who have eating disorders.

Summary

Compared to psychotherapy, which we will discuss in the next chapter, more patients get well, and more quickly, when they take antidepressants. And, as long as they keep taking their prescribed medications, they remain well longer, too.

How Brain Cells Work

The human brain is a very sophisticated and complex organ made up of billions of cells that can be likened to a generator and transmitter of electrical impulses. The brain carries out its function via the neurons (or brain cells) which communicate with each other every moment of our lives, thereby enabling us to function as human beings. Neurons enable the brain to perform all the functions of thinking, speaking, walking, talking, hearing, and seeing. Neurons also control how we feel, including our emotions and moods. (Fig. 5–2)

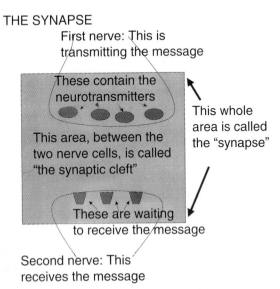

Figure 5–2: The synapse (the space between cells) where neurons communicate with one another.

Neurons communicate with one another via neurotransmitters. These are chemicals that move across the space—the synapse—between cells. (Fig. 5–3) Neurotransmitters function as messengers allowing one neuron to communicate with another cell to perform a certain task. These tasks can be something as simple as making one, or many, muscles contract to make you smile, or frown. The message may be just one of many hundreds sent at the same time to hundreds of other neurons to allow you to perform tasks as complicated as doing long division sums.

A neuron delivers its message by firing an electrical charge—a nerve impulse—along its conducting fiber, the axon. As the impulse moves toward the end of the neuron, it activates tiny reservoirs of chemical neurotransmitters that then travel to the end of the neuron at the synapse. Here, reservoirs are opened, and the neurotransmitters spill into the synapse. One neuron may release several different neurotransmitters at the same time. It is possible, therefore, that serotonin, noradrenaline, and dopamine—all believed to play some role in depression—may be released simultaneously from one neuron.

Neurotransmitters then make their way across the synapse to join another neuron, another cell, at a specific area on its surface. This area can be visualized as a chemical docking station called a receptor site. At the receptor site, the neurotransmitter chemicals are absorbed and are sent to the inside of a receiving cell. Once inside the receiving cell, the neurotransmitters set off another series of chemical processes.

Receptor sites do not process the same neurotransmitter for the same function. Once released by a neuron, a neurotransmitter may head off in several directions to affect different actions. The serotonin receptor site at one location, for example, may be involved in constricting small blood vessels. At another site, a neurotransmitter may be needed to stop

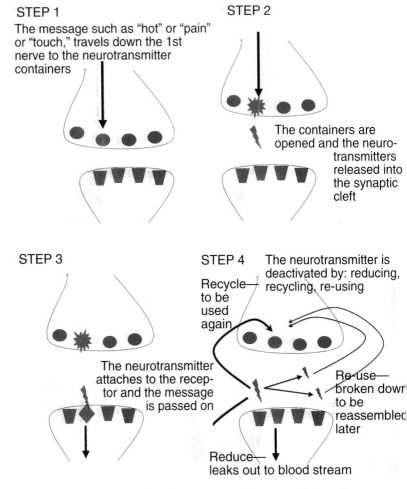

STEP 1

The message such as "hot" or "pain" or "touch," travels down the 1st nerve to the neurotransmitter containers

STEP 2

The containers are opened and the neuro-transmitters released into the synaptic cleft

STEP 3

The neurotransmitter attaches to the receptor and the message is passed on

STEP 4 The neurotransmitter is deactivated by: reducing, recycling, re-using

Recycle to be used again

Re-use—broken down to be reassembled later

Reduce leaks out to blood stream

Figure 5–3: Diagrams showing the sequence of the transmission of a message.

acid secretion in your stomach, or to stimulate specific muscles in your intestine.

The three basic types of neurons are: sensory, motor, and interneurons. Sensory neurons transmit messages to the central nervous system (CNS); motor neurons move messages from the CNS to the muscles or glands; and interneurons, which are located in the CNS, carry all the messages that are transmitted within that system.

As you might expect, all this incessant electrobiochemical activity needs to be regulated. Otherwise, synapses would be flooded, and we might find ourselves endlessly doing the same thing, for example, eating without ever stopping or sitting without ever standing.

Regulation is achieved in several ways. After neurotransmitter(s) are released, a large portion of the substance is taken back, absorbed, and metabolized inside the original firing neuron.

We have described the actions of this very sophisticated, very elegant network of neurons in terms of one neuron sending a message to another. In reality, millions of the billions of neurons, synapses, and neurotransmitters in the human brain are involved, *at the same time in the separate aspects of every simple human activity.* Compared to this, a mainframe computer is a mere toy.

Something as seemingly simple as eating one's breakfast cereal, for example, will involve neurons, synapses, and neurotransmitters that govern senses of sight, smell, touch, and hearing. They will also have something to do with the muscles in your digestive system and with the required physical movements. All will play a role in the release of gastric juices into your stomach, and in your thought processes as you listen to the radio or read the morning paper.

This amazing system works to perfection when you are healthy. However, in the state of depression, the system is malfunctioning, and normal regulation is lost to some small (or large) degree. Some researchers have suggested that in the depressed state,

1. not enough transmitter is being forwarded into the receiving neuron, possibly serotonin and/or norepinephrine and/or depramine

2. the transmitter is not being forwarded into the receiving neuron
3. the receptor sites for the transmitter are not allowing adequate amounts of it to dock.

A fourth possibility is that some critical reaction of which we are still unaware takes place inside the neuron that takes up the transmitter. In other words, it is like a radio with a flat battery—the message is arriving but cannot be heard properly downstream. These downstream effects may turn out to be critical to depressive illness.

Any one of these events, or all four happening together, can result in lower levels of serotonin, norepinephrine, or dopamine. The overall result is a lack of coordination of the brain function. It is like the magnificent orchestra of the brain is without a conductor.

CHAPTER 6

PSYCHOTHERAPY AND OTHER TREATMENTS

Psychotherapy is a method of treating mental and emotional disorders. In psychotherapy, the patient establishes a therapeutic relationship with the therapist (who may or may not be a medical doctor). Within this relationship, all aspects of the illness are discussed. It is hoped that the process will eventually lead to successful treatment of the emotional disorder.

If you are clinically depressed, and choose psychotherapy over drug therapy as a primary treatment option, it may take you a little longer to become well. If you are severely depressed, your chances of a rapid improvement in mood are not as good as with medications. However, the gains made in psychotherapy may last beyond termination of therapy, and there are fewer side effects to psychotherapy.

Psychotherapy enables a different approach to the treatment of depression than medications. Psychotherapy can also help you deal with other issues in your life that may not be a part of the clinical depression—conflicts in your life or in relationships at work are examples.

Many types of psychotherapy are available, but only two have been shown to be scientifically effective for treating mood disorders and depression: cognitive behavioral therapy (CBT) and interpersonal psychotherapy (IPT). Each focuses on the depressive syndrome, and each has an antidepressant action.

Cognitive behaviorial therapy (CBT)

The theory behind this type of therapy assumes that people who are depressed think dysfunctionally. That is, in depressed patients, thinking processes can be distorted and become locked into self-destructive patterns. This kind of thinking can cause the illness or make it worse. The result is distress and the inability to function.

Cognitive behavioral therapy is based on the theory that dysfunctional attitudes precede the development of depression. In other words, dysfunctional attitudes predispose a person to mood disorders. By changing distorted attitudes and by teaching a person how to think differently, depression can be treated and relapses can be prevented.

The following dialogue illustrates the point about distorted thinking:

> George: I've locked my keys in the car again. I'm such a fool. I'm always making these mistakes. I'm pretty useless. My life is pretty meaningless. Why am I bothering about it?
>
> Therapist: Let's identify this thought process. ("I locked my keys in the car. I'm such a fool.") That's what most people say. But you go further. ("I'm always making these mistakes. I'm pretty useless.") Let's look at other alternatives.
>
> How else can you account for locking the keys in the car. Chance? Simple mistake? You were distracted? The next time you leave your car keys locked or make some other mistake, track your thinking. And when you get to the point where you make that leap from feeling foolish like everybody else does, to feeling useless, think about other alternatives.

Cognitive behavioral therapy deals very much with the "here and now." It examines how people view themselves, their relationships with others, and the world at large. The individual is made aware of his or her distorted thinking; he or she then challenges and tries to restructure it. When this is achieved, symptoms of depression fade and then hopefully disappear. The person eventually becomes well.

Cognitive behavioral therapy requires the participant to perform certain tasks and to do homework. Assignments are always chosen with the depressed person's level of dysfunctional thinking in mind. Tasks are selected so that the individual has a good chance of completing them successfully. Success improves the sense of self-worth and esteem and also confronts the depressed person with his or her tendency to set impossible tasks. If people set impossible tasks for themselves, they almost guarantee that a success will never occur. Failure confirms a sense of low self-esteem. "See, I knew I couldn't do it. I'm a failure because I'm no good at anything."

Each CBT session comprises a one-on-one meeting with patient and therapist that lasts up to 1 hour. Some CBT is now offered in a group setting with 6 to 10 other people suffering from depression. During the acute phase of treatment, the sessions are usually held once each week for 20 weeks. During each meeting, therapist and patient examine the latter's thought processes to identify dominant patterns. Once identified, the goal for the client is to change these patterns by considering other alternatives.

Here is an example: A friend declares to a person with depression he cannot go along to a meeting or social event. The depressed person may assume that the refusal means he is not liked by the friend. In CBT, the depressed person is asked to consider other possible explanations for the refusal. Could it be that the friend already has a commitment? Would the friend find the event boring? Is a school or work project to be completed by the next day? Is it possible that this friend is a "fair-weather" friend and only wants to associate with the patient when the depression has lifted? Getting the depressed person to consider other alternatives is the first step in the process of CBT. Next, the person is encouraged to generate possible alternatives right on the spot when the depressing event or interaction taking place.

The best candidates for CBT are those who are motivated and who are psychologically minded, i.e., they believe life events are based on cause and effect, and that often human behavior makes events occur. Good candidates are also motivated to change and able to describe how they are thinking and feeling. Studies show CBT to be effective in 60% of mild-to-moderate depressions. This means CBT is as effective as antidepressants but takes longer—3 to 5 months compared to 5 or 6 weeks with medications. However, unlike the latter, CBT does not produce side effects.

So far, we have no proof that taking antidepressants and following a program of CBT concurrently will allow a depressed person to get better faster. It appears, however, that if patients have symptoms that persist while on medication, these residual symptoms can be improved with CBT.

The practice of CBT is relatively new. It was developed, and its use increased, only within the last 30 years. Not enough therapists with specialized CBT skills are available at this time.

Most CBT therapists are trained psychologists or social workers. Some offer their services at psychiatric departments or clinics. Most work from private offices. Cognitive behavioral therapy provided by other than physicians is not covered under any provincial healthcare plans. However, it may be offered under the terms of some individual or company health insurance policies.

Interpersonal Therapy (IPT)

This type of therapy is newer than CBT. It is based on the principle that dysfunctional relationships exist whenever a depression occurs. The depression itself is not necessarily a direct result of these problems in relationships. The focus of IPT is to work on malfunctioning relationships and to improve them. By doing so, the illness is improved.

"Common sense put into a manual" is one description applied to IPT. Treatment with IPT can be used for both depressive syndrome and depressive symptoms in the young, the elderly, and the physically or medically ill.

Interpersonal therapy has three phases. The first is the *data gathering* phase. This phase begins with a thorough psychiatric evaluation. The evaluation focuses on the current relationships in the patient's life. In particular, the focus is on

What happens if you stay onmedications, or try switching to psychotherapy, or come off medication altogether?

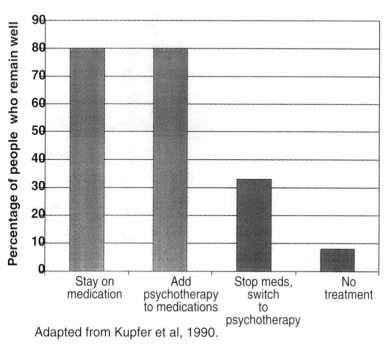

Adapted from Kupfer et al, 1990.

Figure 6–1: Chances of staying well if you stop taking antidepressants.

recent events that have affected relationships—loss, conflict, change, etc.

The second phase *examines and assesses significant relationships* in four major areas, focusing on people's "roles" or the expectations they have or others have of them (Fig. 6–1).

1) Loss
2) Conflicts
3) Change in role
4) Difficulty making or keeping relationships

While working with the patient, the therapist suggests new activities and new relationships as a means to conquer loss or grief. Disputes are examined and discussed, and the patient is prompted to try to resolve them.

The same approach is taken to problems that have arisen from major life changes (e.g., a job change or a move to another town or city). At the same time, efforts are made to improve a patient's social skills.

The third and final phase involves *consolidating progress* which sums up the progress made during previous sessions.

To test the possible benefits of IPT, one study looked at patients who had been taking antidepressants for at least 6 months and were well (Fig. 6–1). Patients were placed in one of three groups. The first group continued with medication; the second was given IPT; the third received a placebo, which is a chemically inert substance that has no specific effect on the mind or body.

After 3 years, 80% of the patients taking antidepressants remained well; 33% of the IPT patients were still well, but only 8% of the placebo group reported they were well. In other words, 92% became sick once more when they stopped taking medication.

Since IPT is still new, there are not many clinicians trained in this form of therapy, but the numbers are growing. The typical program comprises a one-hour session each week for 12 to 16 weeks. When it is provided by a physician, IPT, like CBT, is covered by provincial healthcare plans. Most therapists deal with relationships even if they are not specifically trained in IPT.

Psychodynamic Psychotherapy

Psychodynamic psychotherapy deals with past and present relationships and events. In this type of therapy, patients examine their thoughts, emotions, and behavior throughout their lives. Patients are encouraged to link their thoughts and their emotions, and they are encouraged to look at those parts of their personalities which may cause conflict within themselves and with others.

Treatment sessions in psychodynamic therapy are held once or twice a week. Therapist and patient sit face to face at opposite sides of a desk or table. Sessions may also be held for couples or groups. Psychodynamic psychotherapy is often helpful in cases of mild or moderate depression although studies have not been done to confirm this.

Psychoanalysis

Psychoanalysis involves a journey into the patient's past. The journey is into childhood, where the patient's current mental health problems may have their roots. This is a very intensive kind of therapy that may require daily sessions with a therapist.

In psychoanalysis, the goal is to work back in time through conflicts, emotions, and relationships until the patient finds the core of his or her personality. The patient often, but not always, lies on a couch, talking freely in an attempt to understand his or her emotions during the process of growing up. Meanwhile, the analyst sits behind the patient, out of view, while taking notes and making comments.

Like psychodynamic psychotherapy, psychoanalysis has not yet been scientifically proven to be effective in treating mood disorders and depression. Both may be effective therapies, however, for a variety of life problems or conflicts.

In severe depression, our advice is to try the antidepressants first. In mild or moderate cases, we discuss the benefits and disadvantages of other options with our patients, and we decide together which treatment will be best in each particular case. In two-thirds of cases, antidepressants improve symptoms; the physical symptoms are usually the first to improve followed by the mood symptoms. When patients have recovered, often they feel more desire and have more psychological energy for the work required by psychotherapy.

Other Treatments

Together, you and your doctor may decide that some type of therapy, other than those we have already discussed, may be helpful in treating your depression. Several are available for consideration. Most can be used in all types of depression.

1. Electroconvulsive Therapy (ECT): Electroconvulsive therapy used to be known as "shock treatment," is a treatment that produces seizures by delivering a brief electrical impulse to the brain. The therapy acts at the synapse, just as do antidepressants. There can be no doubt about the effect of ECT which is a most successful treatment for depression, and it relieves all types, particularly psychotic depression.

Electroconvulsive therapy may be the quickest way to relieve depression. If you are depressed and decide on this form of treatment, you will probably undergo two to three ECT procedures per week and receive a total of six to twelve treatments. You will probably have recovered by the end of this 4- to 5-week course, which is in contrast to the 6 to 8 weeks needed with antidepressants.

When introduced in the 1930s, ECT was the only treatment available for depressive illness. At this time, antidepressants had not been developed. Treatments such as insulin coma and hydrotherapy were introduced after ECT, but they failed to help patients who were suffering from major depressions, and these have long since been discarded.

When ECT was first used 60 years ago, it was crude by today's standards. Even then, although quite stressful for patients, it was effective. Patients were awake during the procedure. The high intensity electrical stimulus was delivered through electrodes placed on both sides of the head. The stimulus produced seizures and violent muscle contractions so that patients needed to be restrained during the procedure.

In earlier years, the side-effects of ECT were significant. One was loss of memory. Because of significant side effects, ECT was used less and less frequently through the years. Eventually it was performed only on individuals who failed to respond to all other treatments.

In recent years, however, the technical aspects of ECT have been much improved. Today, patients receive ECT while under a general anesthetic. Muscle relaxants are also used to avoid the violent muscle contractions. The charge is delivered through one or two electrodes. The seizure lasts only 20 to 40 seconds. The patient usually wakes up within 1 minute of the stimulus. If being treated as out-patients, patients may go home or return to work after the session.

Improvements in ECT therapy have reduced the number and severity of its side effects. If you are depressed and agree to have ECT, you may still experience some memory loss for a short time. You may not be able to recall events that happened during the period of ECT therapy. In all other respects, however, you will think as yourself and act as you usually do. For the 3 months following ECT therapy, you may find it difficult to remember details such as the postal code of your last address, or your neighbor's maiden name. But once you check the postal code and the name, you will be able to retain them again.

In fact, 6 months after your last ECT session, you probably will not experience memory loss. Changes in memory and concentration are often a result of depression, and you may find that when your depression lightens, as a result of the ECT, your memory is improved.

Unfortunately, in most cases, the benefits of ECT last for only 4 to 6 weeks; it must be followed by a maintenance program. After ECT treatment is finished, you will likely be put on a schedule of antidepressants. If you and your doctor agree, you can follow a maintenance course of ECT. Treatments may be recommended as frequently as once a week or once a month.

2. Augmentation Strategies: Augmentation refers to a strategy in which one substance is added to an antidepressant that has been used alone and which has not successfully controlled the depressive episode. In most cases, the second agent is not an antidepressant, but when used in tandem with a true antidepressant will prove to be more effective than the antidepressant used alone. Augmentation agents include hormones, amino acids, and psychostimulants. Some examples follow:

- **Thyroid Hormone:** Thyroid hormone can enhance the effect of an antidepressant drug. The thyroid gland, which is located at the front of the neck produces two hormones—T_3 and T_4. Together, these hormones regulate the body's metabolism and temperature among other things.

  If an antidepressant does not appear to be working, a doctor may suggest that a patient take T_3 along with the prescribed antidepressant medication. This has the effect of kick-starting the antidepressant into action. The tactic works with all types of antidepressants and also for patients with normal thyroid function. In 60% of cases, the patient's mood and behavior will improve within 2 to 3 weeks.

- **Lithium:** Used alone, this drug is the preferred treatment for bipolar depression. As a sole agent in unipolar depression, it may prove no better than a placebo. It is particularly effective when used as an augmenting agent in unipolar depression; it helps 55 to 65% of patients.

- **Tryptophan:** This is one of 20 natural amino acids that are involved in the synthesis of proteins in the human body. Tryptophan is also a manufactured synthetic drug that can induce sleep. Like T_3 and lithium, tryptophan boosts the action of some antidepressant drugs.

- **Psychostimulants:** Amphetamines and other psycho-stimulants are sometimes used, but there is little evidence that they are as effective as T_3 and lithium. In addition, they are sometimes addictive.

- **Buspirone:** This is a newer drug that, when used alone, has a mild antidepressant effect. But, like lithium, it is most effective when used in combination with an anti-depressant, especially the SSRIs.

- **Estrogen:** Studies have shown that, in depression, estro-gen will benefit as many as one-third of patients, mostly women. This success rate is not much better, however, than that usually achieved with a placebo. Nevertheless, some patients do feel better on estrogen.

3. Anxiolytics: These drugs are also used as agents to reduce anxiety. They include the benzodiazepine family (e.g., diazepam, lorazepam), which work well to reduce symptoms of anxiety and to help depressed people to sleep. Some depressed people may take anxiolytics to overcome the side effects of antidepressants. In the long term, however, these agents may bring on depressed moods and make depression more difficult to treat in some individuals. Anyone taking an anxiolytic may also need higher and higher doses of the same drug if they develop a tolerance to it. However, if you are taking these drugs, and they are effective, there may be no need to alter the regimen.

4. Light Therapy:

Doctors prefer to use light therapy for patients who suffer from seasonal depression. Light is delivered in one of two ways: through a light box or via a cap or visor (Fig. 6–2). Transmitted light is measured in a unit of illumination called a *lux*. No one knows yet how many lux are needed for the best effect. The number delivered ranges between 60 and 10,000 lux. Most treatments are of 30 to 60 minutes in duration.

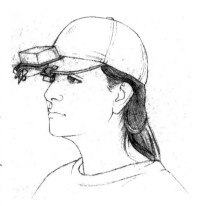

Figure 6–2: Light therapy can be delivered via a cap.

Light therapy helps more than 50% of people who suffer from seasonal depression. Because light therapy acts quickly, the benefits are soon experienced, sometimes within the first week. If a patient's morale does not improve, or if the symptoms do not fade within 2 weeks, light therapy is usually judged ineffective and other treatments are started.

Generally, the side effects of light therapy are not serious: headache, eye strain, a sense of feeling wired, and nausea. Very few people quit this treatment because of side effects. In fact, most patients who suffered from headaches before therapy report an improvement after light therapy.

In most cases patients are exposed to light sources every day for 2 weeks. The optimal time is early morning, upon awakening, for 30 to 60 minutes. Light therapy does not deliver the same kind of light used in tanning salons, where ultraviolet (UV) light is allowed to reach your skin. In light therapy, the UV is blocked. While the box unit can be built at home, it is a job best left to a professional, who can ensure proper light intensity and wiring.

If you think light therapy would help you, talk to your doctor. An advantage of this therapy is that amounts of light can be adjusted as needed. Adjustment may involve the time of day (morning and/or evening); amount of illumination (brightness); and/or exposure (minutes). This is something you and your doctor can decide together. Alternatively, you can check in your local library or phone book for sources of information. Possibly, local experts may be available or you can check with the Society for Biological Rhythms and Light Therapy (www.websciences.org/sltbr/).

5. Experimental Treatments: Several alternative medicinal preparations for depression have emerged recently. Most of these preparations are very unlikely to have any effect. However, many in fact do have pharmaceutical properties. These properties may be beneficial or harmful directly, or may be harmful because they interact with other medicines a person is taking. While there are often enthusiastic claims for the success of these therapies, there is virtually no experimental evidence that they have benefits and no documentation of their potential to cause harm.

There are exceptions. An example of a herbal remedy that is known to have some antidepressant effects is St. John's Wort. There is evidence that, when used as a pharmaceutical preparation (i.e., Hypericum), it is more effective than placebo (or sugar pill) in mild depression and it is perhaps as effective as low-dose standard antidepressants.

However, it has not been demonstrated to be effective in moderate or severe depression, nor has it been shown to have an effect lasting beyond several weeks. What is also a concern is that some of the ingredients in St. John's Wort have the potential to cause serious reactions when mixed with other drugs.

Therefore, St. John's Wort cannot yet be recommended as a treatment for depression because there are better "first line," "proven" conventional medicines. Also, it is important to remember that medicinal herbal or other treatments are not regulated or standardized. Therefore, one cannot be sure that the ingredients listed or the dosages provided are correct.

Whether it is conventional or alternative therapy, you need to know as much as possible about the treatment before you begin. It is important to ask your practitioner about the care he/she is recommending. When asking about a treatment, you should feel that your practitioner is knowledgeable and open to discuss what is known and unknown, good and bad about the treatment. Be suspicious of practitioners who make absolute statements to the effect that treatments are 100% effective or entirely free of side effects. Such treatments do not exist!

Here are some questions to ask your practitioner.

1. What is the evidence that this treatment is effective? Are there scientific studies? Are these "controlled" studies or merely reports of a few successful "cases?"

2. How many patients has the practitioner treated with this therapy? What has been the success rate?

3. If "booster" treatments are being suggested, have they been shown to work with the antidepressant you are taking?

4. What side effects does the treatment have? Which ones are temporary and which remain as long as you take the treatment? Is there a risk of any permanent side effects that might not resolve even if the treatment is discontinued?

5. What are the possible interactions between this drug and other medicines you are taking (including over-the-counter drugs such as cough and cold remedies, "painkillers," contraceptives, etc.)?

6. What are other possible treatments?

6. Neuroleptics: These are major tranquillizers, which are antipsychotic medications given in additon to antidepressants in cases of psychotic depression.

MANAGING DEPRESSION

The majority of depressed people do not receive adequate treatment. Studies have shown that many physicians prescribe antidepressants in doses that are too low and for periods that are too short.

Depression is not always recognized by professional people. Even when it is, treatment rules are not always clear or known.

We emphasize once again that treating depression is a partnership between patient and doctor. It is important that both assume their roles and responsibilities from the start. If you think you may be depressed, one of your responsibilities is to report all the signs and symptoms (see Chapter 2) when you see a doctor for the first time. If you say only that "I always feel tired," your chances of getting an early and correct diagnosis are limited. Fatigue is a common symptom in many illnesses—from workplace burnout to cancer. The doctor must consider other causes of fatigue and be aware of other symptoms if depression is to be diagnosed early.

It may be difficult for a patient to report all the signs and symptoms because they are so elusive. Still, the effort should be made. Your physician should also make some inquiries about your emotional well being that will help you to describe your symptoms. Making a correct diagnosis is the first and most important step in the management of every illness.

Once a diagnosis of depression is made, you and your doctor can discuss the available treatments. Antidepressants and psychotherapies (see Chapter 6) are the most likely options.

Major depression is a chronic, recurrent disorder. If not treated, the illness may worsen and can become chronic. This is why treatment with antidepressant medications must proceed aggressively. We do this by prescribing the highest dose of antidepressant that a patient can tolerate over an appropriate period. If the first medication does not work, we try a second. And, if necessary, a third and a fourth or more. In fact, in our practices, people who come for advice on treatment have already tried an average 8 to 12 different treatments for their depression. Treatment is usually divided into three phases: acute, continuation, and maintenance.

Acute Phase

The acute phase of treatment of depression goes on for as long as it takes to erase symptoms and restore a patient as closely as possible to his or her regular daily activities. Only then can the acute phase of therapy be said to have been completed. In most cases, this phase lasts for 3 months at most. In others it may take longer.

The acute phase of treating depression requires that you and your doctor work together to select the antidepressant that works best. This involves working together to determine the most effective dosage for the appropriate length of time. This period usually lasts 4 to 6 weeks. Although the medication may begin to have an effect around day 10 to 14 of treatment, you need to give it 4 to 6 weeks to work. If you stop taking the medication too soon, you may harm yourself in two ways: you take away the opportunity to get well, and you waste valuable time.

The two most common valid reasons for giving up on an antidepressant are either it is not working for you, or you cannot tolerate its side effects. All antidepressants have side effects. In fact, all medications do, including headache remedies like aspirin. However, side effects usually dissipate after a few weeks. The newer agents, like the selective serotonin reuptake inhibitors (SSRIs), have fewer and milder side effects.

In many cases, it is side effects that prompt people to stop taking the medications. If you are tempted to stop taking a prescribed drug, talk to your doctor. There are some simple interventions that will help relieve most of the common side effects. If a drug is not working, it is important to be sure you have been taking it in prescribed doses for the appropriate period of time.

If you cannot tolerate one drug, it does not mean that you will not tolerate a second, or a third. If you and your doctor decide to give up on one medication, it is important to select a replacement. This policy is not unique to depression. We do not tend to give up on antibiotics if penicillin is not working for an infected throat. Your doctor would prescribe another antibiotic.

The second antidepressant your doctor prescribes may be in the same chemical class as the first. With the tricyclic antidepressants (TCAs) and monoamine oxidase inhibitors (MAOIs), however, the chances that this strategy will work are only about 30%. Switching to another class of drugs increases your chances to 65%. This is almost the same as it was for the drug that was selected first.

With SSRIs, the strategy may be different. To improve your chances of a cure, you need not switch to another class of drugs. If you stop taking the first SSRI and switch to a second, the likelihood of success is almost the same as it was with the first—about 50 to 60%.

Patients should not be necessarily satisfied if they consider a medication is producing only a partial response. If a major symptom, such as having suicidal thoughts is relieved but other symptoms persist just as strongly, you are making progress, but not enough. The chemical abnormality in your brain may not be fully resolved.

One well-known psychiatrist has said, "depression begets depression." What he meant by this is that in some people depression is a progressive disease. Untreated in these people, depression can go from bad to worse.

If a partial response to a medication does not become complete over a certain time period, the medication can be judged ineffective. You and your doctor then have four options. These are:

- increase the dose
- change to another antidepressant
- add an agent that will also work as an antidepressant when used in combination with the existing drug (augmentation)
- use two active antidepressants together.

Continuation Phase

The goal in this second phase of treatment is to prevent symptoms from returning—to prevent a relapse. This means you must continue to be treated even when you are well. If treatment for a mood disorder is discontinued too soon—before 6 months—a patient's risk of becoming ill again soars. If discontinued at 6 months, the patient has a 10% chance of relapse by the end of the year. If discontinued after 3 months, the chance of relapse is 80%.

Six months of antidepressant therapy is not a number pulled out of a hat. For most patients, depression lasts from 6 to 9 months. A 6-month period is usually enough to help patients through the cycle of a biological depression. After that, the illness fades and goes into remission. Usually, patients we see for the first time have been ill for some time. By treating them with antidepressants for another half year, we help them get through the natural course of the illness. If you have had several episodes or severe episodes, you may need maintenance therapy. Figure 7–1 shows the severity of symptoms during onset of depression and its treatment over a period of 6 months. This is discussed in the next section.

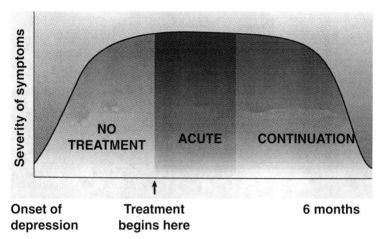

Onset of   **Treatment**   **6 months**
depression   **begins here**

Figure 7–1: It takes time for depression to be cured. This graph shows how antidepressants help control the severity of symptoms over the natural course of the ilness.

Maintenance Phase

Depression has a tendency to return. It can strike again and again. This is especially so in people who have had two or more previous episodes. Most of these patients opt for maintenance doses of antidepressants for an indefinite period. In some cases this could be for a lifetime.

Statistics show why this is necessary. If your present depression is the first in your life, the likelihood that it will recur is slightly less than 50%. If it is your second illness, the likelihood is between 50 and 90%. More than three episodes increase the chances of having yet another episode to greater than 90% (Table 7–1).

Table 7–1: Recurrence of depression	
Number of episodes	% recurrence
1	< 50%
2	50–90%
3 or more	> 90%

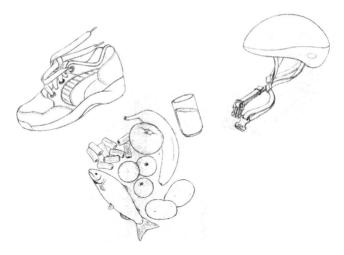

Figure 7–2: It is important to maintain a good diet and regular exercise when depressed as this will likely improve treatment outcome.

Other situations make lifetime drug therapy a possibility. For example, if you have two bouts of illness within a short period of time, or if you have experienced a single episode with a severe consequence, such as a serious suicide attempt, you and your doctor may agree that maintenance treatment is required. An effective dose is one that has just improved your mood. In other words, "the dose that makes you well, keeps you well." There are only a very few good reasons for reducing the original dose required for recovery from the acute phase in this maintenance phase. These include the persistence of side effects, the occurrence of new side effects, or the presence of some new illness.

Exercise, Diet, and Mood

It may be a "motherhood and apple pie" statement to say that to maintain good health, you should eat a well-balanced diet and exercise regularly. Generally, exercise and diet are also important when you are ill (Fig. 7–2).

When a sick person is suffering from a serious mood change, following good advice is not always easy. Some individuals are willing to exercise and do so; others are not, and do not. If depressed people are encouraged to begin exercising, and they stop because of loss of interest or for any other reason, feelings of low self-esteem and uselessness will be reinforced.

Exercise is helpful in depression because when combined with an appropriate diet, it helps prevent weight gain. Weight gain can occur either as a result of the symptoms or as a result of the treatment. Exercise may also help people lose the weight they may have already gained.

Thirty percent of depressed people put on weight as part of their illness, and being overweight only deepens a patient's sense of poor self-esteem. In addition, some medications used to treat depression tend to promote weight gain—particularly, TCAs and MAOIs.

Exercise may also promote self-esteem. This is something you may have tried, or may want to try. Exercise will not necessarily directly improve your mood disorder, but you may find it offers a valuable distraction and a brief relief from some of the symptoms.

Whether you exercise or not, a good diet is essential, even if you are depressed and have a poor appetite. Plenty of scientific evidence shows that certain nutrients, minerals, and vitamins are important in regulating moods.

Tryptophan is useful in depression. Freely available in milk and other dairy products, L-tryptophan is a building block for proteins and other substances, including neurotransmitters. As we noted earlier, tryptophan is used successfully in some cases of depression when used in combination with an antidepressant; individuals on a diet free of tryptophan may rapidly relapse into depression.

The average North American diet is very nourishing. For the most part, we do not have to worry about our intake of vitamins, minerals, and nutrients, that is, if we maintain a proper diet and eat regularly. An average diet, for example, contains all we need of folate and B_{12}, two closely related vitamins that are found everywhere in the body. Both folate and B_{12} are necessary for general good health. While it is difficult to become deficient in B_{12}, which is stored in the liver for up to 3 years, the situation is different for folate which is particularly important in maintaining mood.

Other B-complex vitamins (thiamine, riboflavin, niacin, pyridoxine, pantothenic acid, and biotin) are needed for cognition and brain function. Whether it is caused by disease, infection, lack of certain drugs or vitamins, or something else, distorted brain function is a risk factor for depression.

There is some evidence to show that calcium and magnesium may play some role in adjusting mood. Calcium is needed for, among other things, transmitting nerve impulses from nerve endings to muscle fibers. Magnesium also helps to transmit nerve impulses. Eggs, fish (bones included), dairy products, and leafy vegetables are the major sources of calcium. Magnesium is found in soya beans, nuts, whole grain cereals, milk, meat, and fish.

Simple carbohydrates (sugars) and complex carbohydrates (starches like pasta) can have different effects on a person's mood. Both may cause mood to dip, the simple carbohydrates causing the biggest drop. This is part of what is called postprandial depression.

Some depressed individuals crave carbohydrates, especially the simple ones found in chocolate products, candy, and ice cream. In some people, the craving is so strong it can be considered a symptom of illness. Eighty percent of people with SAD have these yearnings, but only 15% of those with a depression that is not diagnosed as SAD do. Some antidepressants give you a dry mouth and make you thirsty. To prevent the mood change and the weight gain caused by ingesting simple carbohydrates, it is a good idea to chew sugarless gums and slake thirst with sugarfree drinks. Some drugs may also induce a carbohydrate craving. The older TCAs and MAOIs often do.

Some depressed patients tell us that certain health foods or herbal remedies make them feel better. Our major concern is that a lot of money may be spent on products that may have no proven scientific benefit. Another concern is that they may contain unwanted or unknown ingredients. Unlike many so-called "natural remedies," scientific evidence supports the effectiveness of St. John's Wort or Hypericum in cases of mild to moderate depression.

Some food supplements contain active compounds like steroids and thyroid hormones. These products are not pure herbal remedies. They can be artificially manufactured supplements that may carry a brand name. They can and do interfere with body functions. We recommend that before a patient purchases any of these remedies, he or she should check out the contents. In some cases, this information is not on the label. You may have to consult an expert, or go to the library. If you cannot get adequate information, do not use the product.

This is not to say that all these products do not work. At one time L-tryptophan could only be bought in a health food store. Today it is an active and approved product made by a reputable drug company.

Where to Get Help

There are many individuals, groups, and institutions you can contact if you feel you are experiencing a change in mood, or that you may be suffering from depression. Care must be taken, however. Unfortunately, some organizations that profess to help depressed individuals may not be that helpful. Some may even be out to defraud. However, some organizations do provide a valuable resource and may allow a discussion of your own situation with one of their counsellors.

In addition to these resources, other local mental health facilities and programs are helpful. In many hospitals across the country, out-patient departments have mental health clinics. Psychiatric hospitals are available, some as separate institutes, others as part of a general hospital's operation. Most of them have out-patient and/or emergency psychiatric services.

Your family physician is another source of aid and comfort. Ninety-five percent of all depressed patients are treated by family physicians. If you would prefer a private psychotherapist, you can consult the provincial or local association of psychologists or social workers.

Some sources provide all types of treatment while others may offer only one or two. Not all psychotherapists, for instance, will prescribe antidepressants. The majority prefer not to, some because they are not physicians and do not have the authority. Some treatment units specialize in specific areas of mental health such as mood or anxiety disorders. Our advice is to get as much information as you can before making a choice about treatment.

Emergency Treatment for Depression

Any sudden or unexpected change in a depressed person's emotional state can be an emergency. The most dramatic is the thought or expressed wish to end one's life. This is not unusual. Forty percent of people with a major depression have suicidal thoughts (Table 7–2). (So do many people who are not depressed, including teenagers).

If you are a family member or a friend, how do you determine whether you have an emergency on your hands? If a person is threatening to "end it all," the statement must be taken seriously. The situation is urgent, if the person has previously attempted suicide, has written a note, or has announced how it will be done. If the means are at hand—a

Table 7–2: Risk Factors for Suicide

	High Risk	Low Risk
Age	> 45 years	< 45 years
Sex	Male	Female
Marital Status	Divorced or widowed	Married
Employment	Unemployed	Employed
Interpersonal relationships	Conflict	Stable
Family background	Chaotic or conflict ridden	Stable
Physical Health	Chronic illness, Hypochondriac	Good health, Feels healthy
Mental Health	Excessive drug intake	Low drug use
	Severe depression	Mild depression
	Psychosis	Neurosis
	Severe personality disorder	Normal personality
	Alcoholism or drug abuse	Social drinker
	Hopelessness	Optimism
Personal Resources	Poor achievement	Good achievement
	Poor insight	Insightful
	Affect available or poorly controlled	Affect available and appropriately controlled
Social Resources	Poor rapport	Good rapport
	Socially isolated	Socially integrated
	Unresponsive family	Concerned family

Adapted from Adam K. Attempted Suicide. In: Self-Destructive Behaviour. Psychiat Clin N Am 1985; 8:183.

pistol or rifle in the house—the situation is potentially dangerous.

Whether the depressed person will make the attempt or not depends upon a number of factors. How severe is the depression? Is a recent loss of job or relationship involved? Does the person use alcohol? Does he or she live alone? How strong and compelling are the thoughts of suicide? How dangerous or nearly successful was the last attempt? A recent attempt is the best indication that someone is serious about succeeding this time.

Some depressed individuals—and some who are not—will make a gesture toward ending their lives when, in fact, they have no intention of doing so. The gesture is often an attempt to demonstrate their distress to others; it may also be an attempt to find help.

If you feel suicidal, contact a friend or a professional immediately. They will help to point you in the right direction to receive help to get over it. If you suspect a depressed friend or relative may attempt suicide, act on your suspicions right away. Contact a medical unit such as the emergency room at the nearest hospital, or talk to a healthcare professional such as a doctor, nurse, or social worker. You can try—gently—to convince the depressed individual to seek help immediately. Encourage the person to contact a HELP line or other resource.

Family members or friends sharing the same living space as the would-be suicide may have to take precautions. Knives, guns, and other weapons should be locked away. The medicine cabinet should be emptied of all old medicines and of more recent ones that may be harmful. If necessary, restrict access to the car keys.

If you come upon someone who has just attempted suicide, call an emergency service. This is especially important if you do not have training in first aid or any professional healthcare experience.

Drug Overdose

If the person is conscious, ask what he or she has swallowed. Look around. The drug container or some of its contents may be nearby. Call an emergency service or a poison control center and let those on call know what drug is involved. See that the airway is clear and that the person is breathing.

Cuts and Open Wounds
Apply a pressure bandage to the area to stop bleeding. *Try not to use a tourniquet. It can itself sometimes cause more problems.*

Carbon Monoxide
Protect yourself first. Do not enter the house, garage, or car until a second person is alerted to call for help. If possible, open doors and/or windows first. Get the victim into open air. Turn off the source of the gas, or wait for professional help to do the job.

Drowning
Begin artificial respiration as soon as the person is out of the water. Continue until professional help arrives. Many people in fresh water drownings can be revived when artificial respiration efforts are maintained.

Other emergencies, not as worrisome as suicide, can occur in depressed patients. A panic attack is a temporary emergency that comes upon as many as one-third of people suffering from a major depression (Fig. 7–3). The attack is so intense that the patient thinks he or she is going to die. The symptoms appear suddenly and dramatically: rapid, shallow breathing, chest pains, palpitations, pounding heart, dizziness, sweating, trembling, and faintness are symptoms.

It is important to know the difference between a *panic attack* and a *heart attack*. So, unless you have been in this situation before, the best option is to *get medical attention* for the victim as soon as possible. If you have experience, you will know how to proceed: assure the person that death will not occur. Encourage deep breathing, or ask the victim to breathe in and out of a paper bag. The best long-term therapy to prevent these attacks is antidepressants, anxiolytic drugs, and cognitive behaviour therapy (see Chapters 5 and 6).

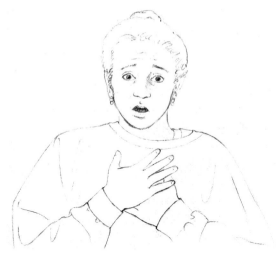

Figure 7–3: A depressed person can experience a panic attack.

It can be considered an emergency if, during a prolonged period of depression, someone decides to stop eating or restricts their food intake to small amounts. Life is endangered here, too, because dehydration and malnutrition can occur. Without adequate food intake, the symptoms of depression will become worse, and physical health will become impaired also. The person could become disabled and no longer be able to, or want to, look after him or herself. Serious, life-threatening medical complications such as heart problems may follow.

In these situations—as a relative or friend—you may have no option but to have the patient assessed in a psychiatric unit. This could prove to be a very unpopular act, but it could be a life-saving measure.

To have a person assessed in a psychiatric unit against their will, you must go before a justice of the peace—not necessarily with the patient—to present the facts of the case. If convinced, the justice of the peace will authorize the assessment. A psychiatrist will evaluate the patient's case, and a decision will be made about hospitalization and treatment.

CHAPTER 8

DEPRESSION AND PREGNANCY

The treatment of a pregnant depressed patient has important considerations for both patient and physician. Decisions have to be made only on the basis of informed choice, after both the pregnant patient and her physician are aware of, and have discussed, all the issues.

If the depression is severe, if the patient does not want to use psychotherapy, or if it has failed to help, antidepressant medications may be considered. However, there may be risks to the fetus when drugs are taken during a pregnancy. There may also be risks to the fetus if the mother remains depressed. These risks must be weighed against each other when making a decision. In our opinion, it is a mistake to decide against using medications without complete knowledge of their potential risks and benefits.

When one of our depressed patients becomes pregnant, our advice is to follow the course that is best for both the mother and the fetus. The decision about the best course of action, however, is not always clear cut and obvious. Many issues must be considered and discussed with our pregnant depressed patients when they are taking antidepressants (Fig. 8–1). The first is the health of the fetus. Human organs form during the first 12 weeks, known as the first trimester

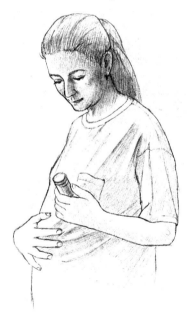

Figure 8–1: Many factors must be considered when taking antidepressants during pregnancy.

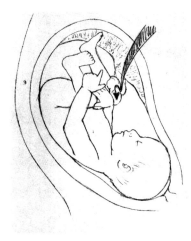

Figure 8–2: Antidepressants can be transferred to your baby through the placenta.

of pregnancy. This is the period when medications are most likely to produce defects. It is also the period when your good health— physical and mental—is important to the developing embryo.

If you are pregnant and have a major depression during this time, it is important that you receive treatment of some kind. Without treatment, your depression may deepen. You may sleep poorly, stop eating, and become malnourished— even suicidal. Any one, and all, of these symptoms are a threat to fetal well being. Taking antidepressants, on the other hand, may also be a risk (Fig. 8–2).

The first months after giving birth can be very stressful, especially if a major depression develops. A new mother may not be able to take care of herself or her newborn child. If a mother made the decision not to receive treatment during pregnancy, she may also decide to continue without treatment. If a profound depression then develops, the baby may be at risk again.

Breast feeding is another issue that should be discussed fully and well in advance of the baby's birth. If you decide to take antidepressants and breast feed, you will essentially be giving these medications to your baby. The choice, then, is between antidepressants and breast feeding. This is not just a medical issue. Currently, for many women breast feeding is an essential component of good childcare.

Table 8–1: Antidepressants that are Safer to Use in Breast-Feeding Mothers		
SSRIs		
Fluoxetine*		
Paroxetine		
TCAs		
Imipramine		
Amitriptyline		
Desipramine		
Nortriptyline		
Doxepin		
Trimipramine		
Clomipramine		
Maprotiline		
Protriplyine		
Amoxapine		
Trazadone		

*Other drugs in this new class of medications have yet to be investigated for their possible use by breast-feeding mothers.

Fortunately, antidepressants are probably among the safest drugs you can take during pregnancy and breast feeding. Studies have shown they do not appear to cause fetal abnormalities. Table 8–1 lists the antidepressants recommended for breast-feeding mothers. The SSRIs fluoxetine and fluvoxamine are the two antidepressants least likely to enter breast milk.

In some cases—and perhaps yours is one—it may not be necessary to take medication during pregnancy. Some depressed women feel better during their pregnancies. Pregnancy sets off a massive change in every woman's endocrine (hormone) system and in the ways the body functions. In some cases, a depressed woman's symptoms and moods may improve.

Overall, there is a balance between the risk of taking medication and the risk of not taking medication. Psychotherapy is a consideration, but remember it may take slightly longer to recover as compared with medication. Whatever you decide, get as much information as you can.

CHAPTER 9

CHOOSING THE RIGHT TREATMENT

Since 1989, many new drugs have become available for treating depression. Although these newer drugs are more specific in their actions than the older ones, all classes of antidepressants work equally well. They differ only in the number and severity of their side effects.

There is a 65 to 75% chance you will get better with the first antidepressant you try. If you are suffering from a severe depression, medications are more likely to help you than psychotherapy. This is why antidepressants are often tried first. In some cases of severe illness (in people who cannot take oral medications, for example), electroconvulsive therapy may be the best first choice. There is some scientific evidence that the tricyclic antidepressants may be slightly more effective for severe cases and that the SSRIs may be slightly better for milder or moderately severe cases.

No one antidepressant is better than the others, but certain antidepressants may be better for certain types of depression. Monoamine oxidase inhibitors (MAOIs), for example, are effective in some cases of atypical depression; MAOIs work well, too, if you exhibit a social phobia or social anxiety as part of your illness. Selective serotonin reuptake inhibitors (SSRIs) also work well in many subtypes of depression, including those that exhibit obsessive-compulsive symptoms and those that have anxiety symptoms and/or disorder, including panic disorder.

The possibility of side effects—the side-effect profile—is always considered by physicians before they prescribe any medication. Generally, the newer antidepressants produce fewer side effects. This is a distinct advantage because unpleasant side effects are the major reason patients refuse to take their medications—no matter what the illness.

Some side effects are directly linked to a drug's mode of action, so they are unavoidable. For example, SSRIs produce stomach upset, insomnia, restlessness, and sexual dysfunction. That is because serotonin plays a role in regulating these functions.

When selecting an antidepressant, safety is another important issue. The older agents are not as safe as the newer ones. The margin between the amount of a tricyclic antidepressant (TCA) needed to provide some benefit, and the amount that can produce a toxic, sometimes dangerous, effect, is narrow. By contrast, it takes a very large amount of any SSRI—well above the therapeutic dose—to produce a toxic result.

Another difference between SSRIs and TCAs is in how they affect the heart. TCAs interfere with the electrical conduction that takes place in this vital organ. The newer drugs do not. That is to say that TCAs are just as effective as SSRIs, but they have more troublesome side effects.

Medications do interact with one another, so drug interactions are another consideration. This interaction affects how they work and the results they produce. It is important that you to tell your physician what other drugs you are taking.

The SSRIs are associated with a variety of drug interactions compared to some other antidepressants. They tend to prolong the action of other drugs. For example, the SSRIs may enhance the action, and therefore side effects, of beta blockers (e.g., propranolol), calcium channel blockers (e.g., verapamil), and other drugs. Drug interactions however, are usually easy to manage, provided your doctor knows exactly which drugs you are taking.

When taken with other drugs, MAOIs produce the most interactions. In particular, they produce a terrific, rapid rise in your blood pressure if taken with certain other drugs. The same thing happens when you are using an MAOI and take food or drink that contains the chemical tyramine. Aged cheese, soy products, aged meats and ripe banana peels are examples of food high in tyramine.

If your brother, sister, mother, or father responded to anti-depressant therapy in the past, your chances of doing well on them may be improved. Knowledge of a family history of depression is useful for a physician when making a decision about the type of therapy to advise.

You may find that your physician prefers one medication and you another. Making a choice is not always easy. Physicians may favour one drug because they have used it often, and successfully. They are also familiar with its actions and side effects.

You may not always agree with your doctor's choice. Within the terms of a working partnership, you have every right not to. Exercising this right, however, should not become the most important issue in your treatment. It is a matter of maintaining balance. If one partner, or the other, begins to dictate, the working relationship is rapidly destroyed.

CHAPTER 10

YOUR FAMILY, YOUR JOB, AND DEPRESSION

Most psychiatrists believe that each of us is born with a certain vulnerability to depression. However, an individual prone to depression cannot be identified before the first episode of depression occurs. We do not really know why depression occurs in some people and not in others. But, as we discussed in earlier chapters, there is no lack of theories.

Many depressed people try to pinpoint the "cause" of their illness and may cite these triggers as a cause of their depression. Some patients believe that their depression will lift if they remove, or get away from, the cause they have identified. Our advice in these cases is to wait until a treatment has had a chance to work. Deciding, for example, that pressures of work are enough for you to quit your job may turn out to be a hasty, career-ending decision (Fig. 10–1).

A situation is made worse if a patient thinks that a decision to remove a "cause" means medication or other treatment is unnecessary because the cause of the discomfort has been removed. A better strategy is to consider all treatment options regardless of whether or not a cause or "trigger" has been identified. Discuss your plans with your physician, financial expert, and other family members.

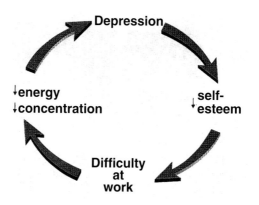

Figure 10–1: The vicious circle of depression: deciding that difficulties at work experienced during an episode of depression are enough for you to quit your job may be a hasty career-ending decision.

Trouble with a family relationship is often cited by patients as a cause of depression. A review of the circumstances, however, usually shows the illness was sometimes in place before the relationship failed. As it continued to fail, the patient felt worse. On the other hand, sometimes disharmony in a family relationship may be the precipitant of a depressive illness. Regardless of the exact timing, treatment can and does help.

Many patients also report that a loss of one kind or another is the reason for their depression. The various types of losses are discussed in Chapter 6. It is good to be aware that some losses can occur in positive circumstances. A job change may be considered a loss because fellow workers and friends may be left behind.

What Can Family Members Do?

If your wife, husband, or partner is suffering from depression, it is essential that you and every other member of the family successfully manages to get through the illness, too. To accomplish this, the best strategy is to be who you are—wife, husband, partner—and do the things you did before one of the partner became ill.

This does not mean you should ignore or disregard the patient, but it does mean that you avoid becoming "down" or "blue" along with him or her. Treat yourself as you normally would. Go out to the movies, visit friends, go bowling. Do whatever you usually do for relaxation and recreation.

What you should not do is try to become responsible for either the patient's recovery or illness. Major depression, as we have said, sometimes leads to thoughts of suicide. In some situations, this feeling becomes so strong that the attempt is made. It is beyond your capacity and your duties to treat such a patient. Call the patient's doctor, or some other professional individual or organization, to get help. A call for help is not a sign of weakness; it is a sign of great common sense, practicality, and of a realistic approach to a problem.

You may find that help and support are to be found in talking to others who are in similar situations. This will certainly reduce your mental and emotional burden and your sense of isolation. Usually you can contact such people through self-help organizations.

Children are a special concern when one of the parents is ill with depression. It is best that children be protected from the illness; however, that does not mean that they have to be protected from the parent with the illness. This, of course, is a big job, especially when younger children are involved who are more dependent upon their parents. You will have to be a very active parent to succeed. But you must do your best to try to keep young children far away from as many aspects of the illness as you can. As much as possible, a child's daily life should remain the same as before the illness occurred. Encourage and give children permission to do what growing, healthy children like to do. All of these steps are intended for one purpose—to keep the child in the world of the child, away from the domain of depression, but not necessarily away from the depressed parent.

If the child is mature enough, education about depressive illness may be of great help. Help may be available through readings, if they are age-appropriate; mental health workers; or through self-help groups. The important point is that help for a child must be appropriate to the child's age group. A 3-year-old child might be told "mommy is not well right now," whereas a 10-year-old may be able to handle information about the depressive illness. The choice of words and concepts to be explained depends on an individual child's level of maturity. It is important, however, to ensure that the child does not take on, or feel, any responsibility for the onset of the depressive illness or the management of a parent's condition.

COMMON QUESTIONS AND ANSWERS

Q: I often feel depressed. Does this mean that I am really ill?
A: All of us can feel depressed at times about things that happen in our lives, but clinical depression is more than just a feeling state. It really is an illness. While it may occur after a stressful event or "out of the blue" a depressive episode may not be due to any specific cause. Being depressed does not mean you have a weak character or that your personality is flawed in any way. Depression can happen to anybody, in any group or class, in any culture or country.

Q: Are my children more likely to become depressed because I am?
A: Depression is not a contagious illness. Your children cannot catch it from you. But since genetic factors play some part in this illness, your children are more liable than other young adults to become depressed *later on when they are adults*. Even so, the chances of this happening are not much greater than they are for any other child. If any symptoms of depression were to appear some years from now, when your son or daughter is an adult, it is quite likely that better medications, psychotherapies, and other treatments will be available for them.

Q: Is there a blood test or something like an x-ray to show if I'm really ill with a depression?
A: No, there isn't yet for primary depression. A lot of research is underway, however, to provide more information about the biology of depression. Early evidence suggests that the newer brain imaging technique may help us to identify some abnormalities. But this technique is in the very early stage of its development and is not used just yet in everyday practice.

Q: Will my depression go away on its own? Do I really need to be treated?

A: Depression, generally, is an illness that comes and goes. So there is a chance that if you wait long enough, it will go away and you will feel better, but you might have to wait for months or years for this to happen. Depression is a serious illness that can become worse. It can have a terrible impact upon your family, your work, and the quality of your life. It is important to get treatment early so it will not get worse or become chronic. The sooner you get treatment, the sooner your symptoms will go away and the sooner your suffering will end.

Q: How long do I have to take my antidepressant medication?
A: Generally, it takes about 6 weeks for an antidepressant to improve your symptoms. It may take a bit longer if the first one does not work and you switch to a second. Once your symptoms have lifted you should stay with your medication for another 6 months. This will greatly reduce the chances of your symptoms returning. Eventually you and your doctor will have to decide whether you should continue taking your medication even longer to prevent recurrences of the illness. Some people take antidepressants for many years, even for a lifetime. This is particularly true if people have had many previous episodes of depression (Fig. A).

Q: Are anti-depressants addictive?
A: No, they are not. They are not street drugs. They do not make you "high" or artificially elevate your mood. Unlike addictive drugs,

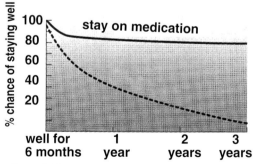

Figure A: Percentage chance of staying well if you keep taking your medication compared with going off it.

which have immediate impact, antidepressants may take 3 to 4 weeks to work. When the time is right and the depression is under control, some people may stop taking their medication. If the drug is withdrawn too quickly, some physical symptoms may occur, but these symptoms will disappear after a day or two. If they have another episode of depression and have to start taking medication again, some of them think this could be a sign of addiction. Taking antidepressants or other medications for depression is not a sign of addiction, it merely indicates that medications are needed. People suffering from diabetes need insulin to stay well. This is not to say that they are addicted to insulin, only that insulin is necessary for them to live a normal life.

Q: Are the side effects I am getting now from my antidepressants permanent?
A: Side effects can be troublesome at first, but for the most part they are not dangerous. The newer antidepressants, like the SSRIs and the mixed reuptake inhibitors, have fewer and milder side effects, and they will often disappear after a few weeks of treatment (Fig. B). There are no lasting effects from antidepressants. Once you stop taking them, your body eliminates them from your system, and the side effects disappear.

Q: Should I change my lifestyle because I am depressed?
A: It is not a good idea to make important life decisions while you are suffering an episode of depression.

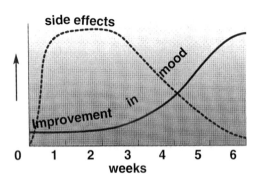

Figure B: Side effects of the newer antidepressants often disappear after a few weeks.

Some decisions such as closing a mortgage cannot be postponed or delayed. You should, however, postpone any other major decisions that do not have deadlines because your memory, your concentration, and your ability to make decisions may not be at their best. You should also understand that a big change in your lifestyle—a change in job or partner, for example—is not likely to improve your depression. You can still, however, make minor changes to your lifestyle; diet and exercise are examples.

Q: What should I do if I feel like killing myself?
A: This is a very common feeling among people who are depressed. It is not unusual because it is part of the syndrome of depression. Ideally, you should have worked out a plan to get help and support *before* you feel the urge to act upon this feeling. Once you feel the need to act, you can call upon the emergency department of the nearest hospital, your doctor, the local crisis line, or a friend as a best source of immediate help. Suicidal thoughts are part of the illness of depression. They will go away once the symptoms are treated.

Q: My doctor and I agreed I should try a different medication, but I notice the dose is different. Also, why don't I have to take this one as often as the first?
A: To achieve their effects, one of the things drugs have to do is get into and stay in your bloodstream at a certain critical level. Some drugs are stronger or more potent than others. You will probably need less of the stronger drugs to reach this critical level. Drugs stay in the bloodstream for different periods of time before they are eliminated. Quickly elimiated drugs need to be taken more often than those that are only slowly eliminated.

Q: I really start to feel bad at about ten o'clock every morning. Does depression always occur at a certain time of the day?

A: Many depressed people have what is known as diurnal variation. This occurs when you feel more depressed in the morning but feel better as the day goes on. Some depressed people feel better in the morning and worse as the day progresses—reverse diurnal variation—but there aren't as many of these latter cases. Despite the fact that your mood changes, you still may be suffering from a major depression.

Q: Should I be concerned that my depression is making me an unfit parent?

A: Your illness means your partner or helpers will have more to do for the children. This is unavoidable. It is most likely to be temporary because your illness can be treated, and you can become well again. You may feel you are not doing a good job as a parent, but we have found that many patients actually continue to do a good job as parents. They are able to perform various duties and handle some responsibilities in a reasonable way. Depressed people just do not feel that they are doing well, although they often are.

Q: If I am depressed, is there any hope for me?

A: Yes, there is. And plenty of it. People with depression do get better. They can and do conquer the illness. That is one of the things that makes treating these men and women such a rewarding part of medicine. It is both a privilege and a very satisfying experience to help people return from a serious, major depression to good health, often within 3 months. The outlook for people suffering from depression is bright in terms of better medications and other therapies, today and in the future.